THE CELLULAR HEALTH DIET GUIDEBOOK

Harness the Power of Your Cells for Energy, Vitality, and a Longer Life

DR. MARIA T. SAMUELSON

TABLE OF CONTENTS

INTRODUCTION

UNLOCKING THE POWER OF YOUR CELLS

There is no complicated scientific reason for this term. It simply refers to the condition of your cells. This is a more intriguing way to think about the health of cells:

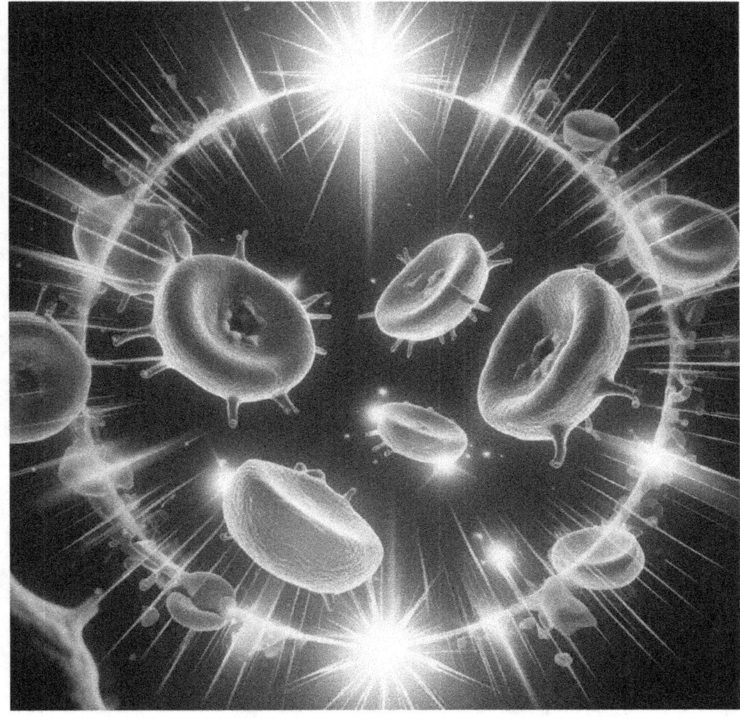

The health of every cell in your body is important for your general, whole-body health. You can conceptualize cellular health as the state of your cells at a cellular level. Since healthy cells work well together, a healthy body is healthier overall. In this way, understanding the health of cells can be both complex and straightforward. This also implies that your actions and participation in health optimization programs can significantly alter the health of your cells. But why is it important for cells to be healthy? It's essential to take care of your cells because they directly impact how your body works, heals, and makes new cells and a lot more. Even more seriously, it's important to understand cellular health because it affects your chances of:

- Getting some genetic diseases.
- Getting cancer as you age
- Having a number of other health problems and diseases

Learning about and taking steps to improve the health of all of your cells is one of the best things you can do to improve your general health, daily energy, and long-term health outcomes. Let's jump right in!

Why Cellular Health Is Important

When people talk about health and wellness, they often talk about things that are outside of themselves, like food, exercise, supplements, or the newest wellness trends. Cellular health, on the other hand, is the most basic idea behind all of these things. At the cellular level, everything in your body starts, from how you digest food to how you think, feel, and even age. Cells comprise your body. In fact, the health of your cells tells you everything you need to know about your general vitality, resilience, and longevity.

Think of your body as a city. Your cells are like the buildings in a city. Building health determines city success, and cell health determines body health. A healthy diet and workout won't matter if your cells are struggling. Your body will still have trouble. The health of cells affects everything, from energy production to immune system function, cleansing, and repair.

Healthy cells, akin to well-maintained buildings, exhibit enhanced resilience against stress, illness, and aging.

It's clear that cellular health is important. The body cannot work right without healthy cells. However, proper cell care can prevent chronic diseases, boost energy, improve cognition, and slow aging. To put it simply, healthy cells are the key to living a long, joyful life.

How Cellular Energy Drives Vitality and Longevity

Energy is a strong force that drives everything we do. It's inside every cell. The majority of this energy originates from microorganisms known as mitochondria, often referred to as the "powerhouses" of the cell. You make adenosine triphosphate (ATP) from the food you eat and the air you breathe. It powers the activities of your cells. Your cells work best when they have a lot of ATP. They can repair themselves fast, get rid of toxins, and adjust to changes in their environment.

There is a catch, though: over time, the mitochondria in our cells start to lose both number and power. This reduction in energy production, known as mitochondrial dysfunction, can lead to fatigue, sluggishness, and an increased risk of illness. In addition to wasting energy, mitochondrial dysfunction speeds up age by making it harder for cells to heal and grow back. In the end, this process speeds up cell damage that leads to a number of long-term health problems, including heart disease, diabetes, and cognitive diseases like Alzheimer's.

Optimizing mitochondrial function and making sure your cells are making enough energy, on the other hand, can make you much healthier and longer-lived. You can keep your mitochondria working well by giving them the right nutrients, lowering reactive stress, and encouraging efficient energy production. This will improve your health as a whole. Your body can work at its best when there is a lot of cellular energy. This keeps you healthy, young, and strong for a lot longer than you might think.

The Link between Cellular Health And Overall Well-Being

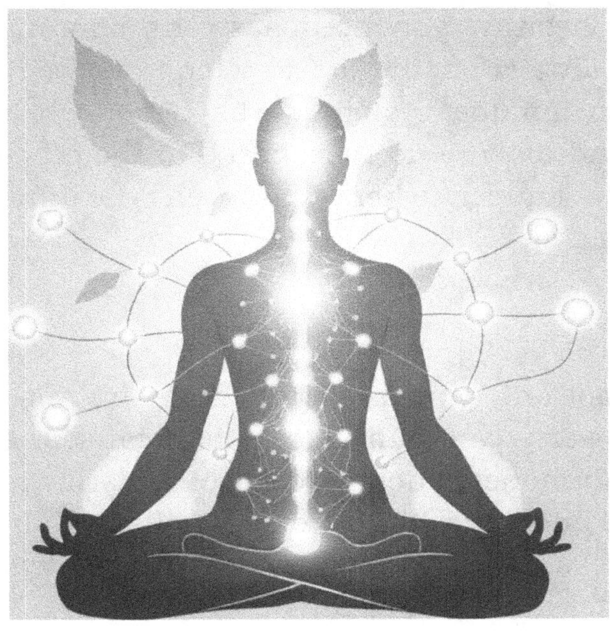

The unseen force that holds your whole life together is your cellular health. It affects how you feel, speed of recovery, and daytime energy. But that's not all—the health of your cells also affects your mental focus, emotional health, immune system, and even the way your skin looks. Here's how your general health directly relates to the health of your cells:

Energy and Vitality

You'll feel worn out and sluggish if your cells aren't making energy properly. You'll have more energy to get through the day if your cells can make more of it. This is true whether you're working hard at work, working out, or spending time with family and friends. You'll feel more alive and interested in life when your physical energy is at its best.

Mental Clarity and Cognitive Function

The billions of cells that make up the brain require a lot of energy to function properly. When your brain cells don't get enough energy or are under too much stress, they lose their ability to think and remember things. In the long run, this can cause brain fog, memory loss, and even more dangerous neurological conditions. Focusing on the health of your cells, especially by optimizing your mitochondria, can help you think more clearly, concentrate better, and keep your brain working well as you age.

Immune System Strength

To fight off infections and stay healthy, you need a strong immune system. Your immune cells are always on the job to keep your body safe from outside threats. Your immune system works better when your cells have enough energy and tools to do their best. On the other hand, immune system problems happen when cells aren't healthy, which makes you more likely to get sick.

Emotional Strength

The health of your cells affects not only your physical energy but also your mental balance. Long-term worry can damage cells and cause the body to make too many stress hormones, such as cortisol. This hurts your mood, your ability to sleep, and your general emotional strength. Focusing on the health of your cells, especially by learning how to deal with stress, can help you feel better and more calm.

Skin Health and Appearance

The cells in your skin are always turning over. Healthy cells are important for making collagen, fixing skin damage, and growing new skin. If your skin cells are not receiving enough nutrients or are overloaded with toxins, it becomes evident. Your skin becomes dull, saggy, and more prone to developing lines. You can keep looking young, have glowing skin, and have a general glow by improving the health of your cells.

What This Book Will Teach You

This book serves as a comprehensive guide to understanding your cells' health, enhancing it, and restoring it. You'll learn about the science behind cellular energy, how your cells work, and why taking care of their health is essential for your general health. But knowing things isn't enough on its own. This book is also full of useful, doable tips that will help you increase the energy in your cells, slow down the aging process, and make you stronger. These tips include:

- **Dietary Strategies for Cellular Health:** Learn which foods are beneficial for your cells, give them the nutrients they need, and make mitochondria work better. To get the most energy and keep your cells healthy, learn how to make a balanced, nutrient-dense meal.
- **Detoxification Techniques:** Learn how to get rid of toxins in your body that can hurt cells and make chronic diseases more likely. Check out some simple and effective detox methods that will clean out your cells and make your body feel better.
- **Making changes to your lifestyle can help your cells heal:** Learn how habits like exercise, sleep, and dealing with stress affect your cells and what you can do to make changes to your lifestyle that help your cells heal and grow.
- **The Power of Movement:** Find out how exercise can improve the efficiency of your mitochondria, give you more energy, and help stop the decline that comes with getting older.

- **Monthly Meal Plan:** An organized, easy-to-follow monthly meal plan will show you the foods and supplements that are good for your cells. This plan will teach you how to eat to get energy, stay healthy, and be strong.
- **Creating a Long-Lasting Routine:** We will provide you with the tools to create a long-lasting health routine that supports your goals for living longer, promotes cell growth, and improves your mood.

You'll know everything and have the tools to improve cell health by the end of this book. It's not enough to just look good; you also need to feel great, have the energy to enjoy life to the fullest, and live a long, healthy life. Taking charge of your health starts with getting your cells to work for you.

PART 1:

UNDERSTANDING CELLULAR HEALTH

<h1 style="text-align:center">CHAPTER 1</h1>

<h1 style="text-align:center">THE SCIENCE OF CELLS – YOUR BODY'S POWERHOUSE</h1>

Trillions of cells in the human body collaborate to sustain our life. These tiny building blocks are in charge of many things in the body, from making energy to fixing tissues and allowing complex processes to happen. Understanding the health of cells is the first step to finding out how to live a long, healthy life. This chapter dives into the fascinating field of cellular biology. It examines the fundamentals of cell construction and function, their energy production and communication, and the impact of cell health on disease and aging.

The Basics of Cell Structure and Function

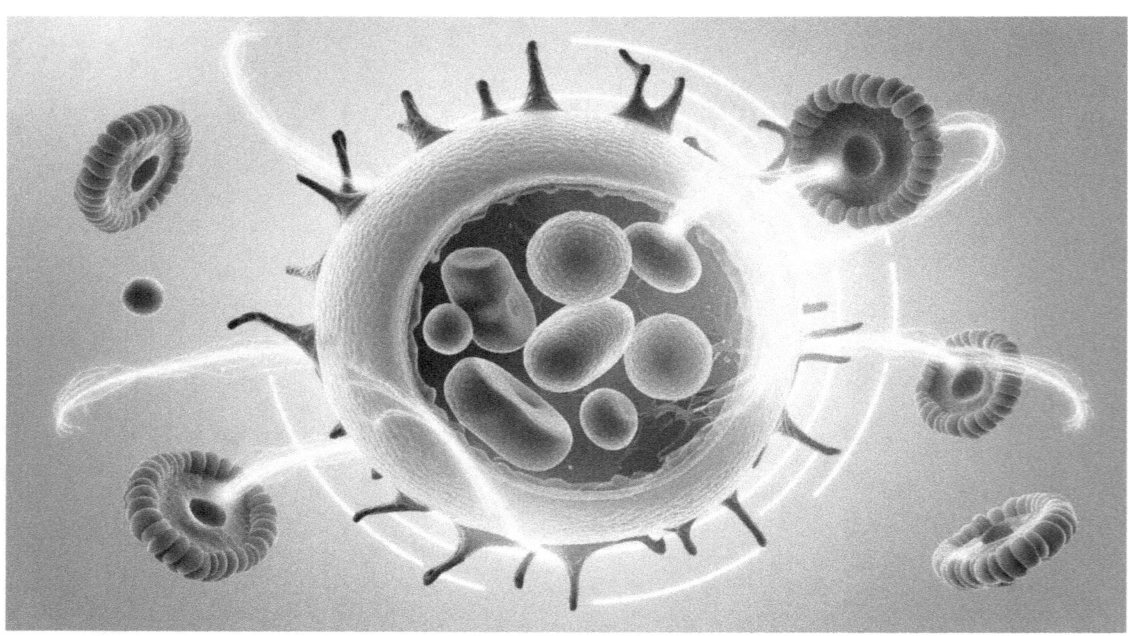

In living things, cells are the smallest functional parts. People often refer to them as the "building blocks" of the body. Each cell is a separate, living thing that can do all the basic things it needs to do:

stay alive, grow, and reproduce. Despite their small size, cells are incredibly complex. They have many different shapes, and each one does a specific job.

The Anatomy of a Cell

A typical human cell consists of three main components:

Cell Membrane

The cell membrane controls what goes in and out of it and keeps it safe. Two layers of phospholipids and proteins make up the membrane, acting as channels, sensors, and enzymes. It is essential for cell health that the membrane can control the uptake of nutrients and the removal of waste.

Cytoplasm

The cell is filled with cytoplasm, a gel-like material that gives organelles a place to move around. It contains water, salts, and various chemical molecules essential for cell function. This is the location where enzyme processes that aid in metabolism occur.

Nucleus

People often refer to the nucleus as the "control center" of the cell because it houses DNA, the genetic code that governs all cellular functions. The DNA code tells the body how to make proteins, which do most of the work inside the body.

Organelles

Organelles, which are specialized parts of cells, have different jobs to do. Among the most important cells are:

- **Mitochondria:** makes energy.
- **Endoplasmic Reticulum (ER):** Makes lipids and proteins.
- **Golgi apparatus:** This part of the cell changes, sorts, and packages proteins for release.

- **Lysosomes:** Break down waste and reuse parts of cells.

The Role of Cells in the Body

To keep balance, cells don't work alone; they work together as tissues, organs, and systems. As an example:

To move, muscle cells have to contract.

Nerve cells talk to each other by sending electrical messages.

Myeloid cells defend the body against germs.

Cells that work well make sure the body can fix damage, fight off illness, and deal with stress.

Cellular Energy: Mitochondria and ATP

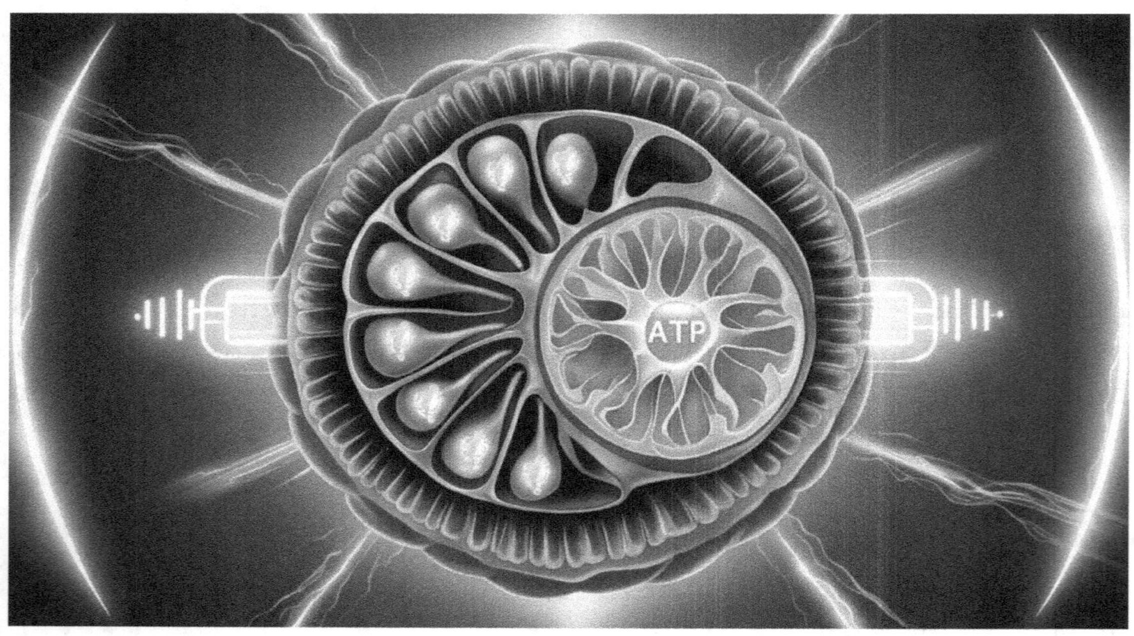

Cells depend on energy to do their jobs. Energy is the coin of life. Cells generate energy through the mitochondria, often referred to as their "powerhouses".

The Role of Mitochondria

Because mitochondria are separate organelles with their own DNA, they can copy themselves without help from the cell. They make adenosine triphosphate (ATP), a molecule that saves energy and releases it when needed, which is the body's main source of energy.

How ATP is Produced

When cells breathe, they go through a set of chemical reactions called cellular respiration. This process has three main steps:

Glycolysis: Carbohydrates break down into glucose in the cytoplasm, which makes a small amount of ATP and pyruvate.

The Krebs Cycle (Citric Acid Cycle): Pyruvate enters the mitochondria and undergoes further breakdown to produce electron carriers in the Krebs Cycle, also known as the Citric Acid Cycle.

The Electron Transport Chain (ETC): is a group of proteins in the mitochondrial membrane that move electrons around. This creates a gradient that powers ATP production.

The body uses this very effective method to turn food into energy it can use. However, damage to mitochondrial function reduces energy production, leading to fatigue, illness, and a compromised immune system.

Mitochondria and Oxidative Stress

Reactive oxygen species (ROS) are byproducts that mitochondria make when they make ATP. ROS help cells communicate and fight off infections when they are present in small amounts. However, excessive ROS can damage certain parts of cells, leading to oxidative stress, a significant factor in aging and chronic illnesses.

How Cells Communicate and Regulate

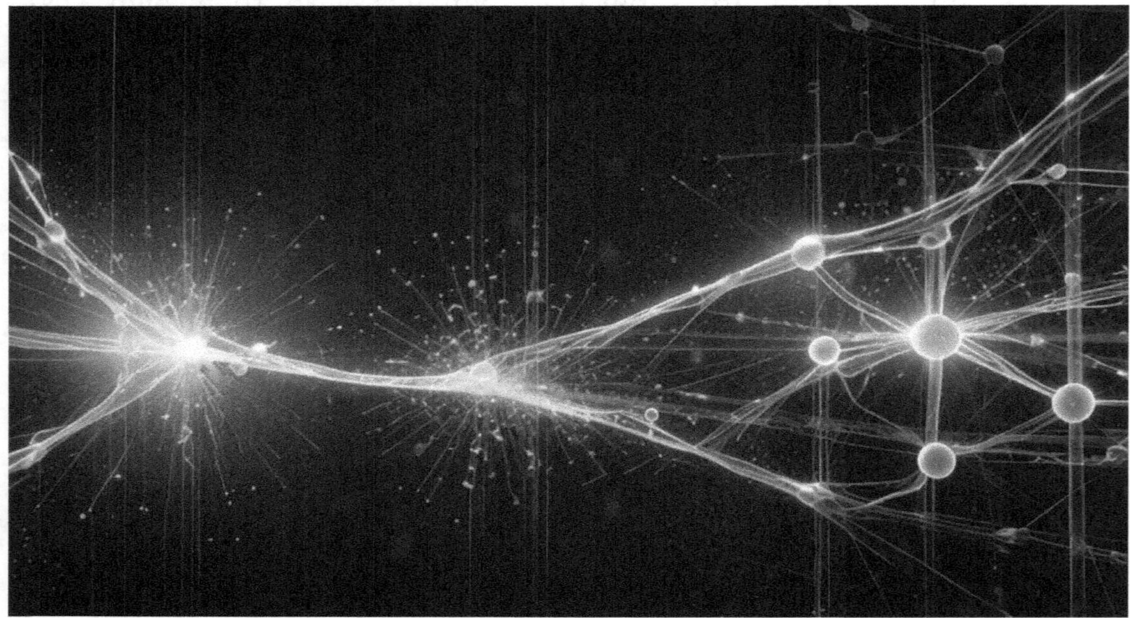

The body functions as a whole due to the complex web of communication that connects all cells. For processes such as growth, repair, immune defense, and maintaining the body's internal environment balance, known as homeostasis, this type of contact is essential. Communication and control between cells use complicated signaling paths, molecular messengers, and feedback systems to make sure cells react correctly to changes in and outside the body. Let's take a closer look at these steps.

Cellular Communication Pathways

Different signaling pathways allow cells to talk to each other. These components of cells enable them to communicate and collaborate to accomplish tasks. Cell phone conversation comes in three main forms:

Autocrine Signaling

An autocrine signal is when a cell talks to itself. It is the cell that sends out the signaling molecules, which then connect to receptors on its own surface.

During an infection, immune cells like T-cells create cytokines that help the body's own defenses work better.

Paracrine Signaling

In paracrine signaling, cells talk to cells nearby by sending signaling molecules into the area around them. The messages only go a short way before they connect with receptors on cells nearby. Neurotransmitters, such as dopamine and serotonin, are chemicals that nerve cells use to talk to nearby neurons or muscle cells.

Endocrine Signaling

Cells release hormones into the bloodstream. These hormones can travel long distances and change cells in other parts of the body. The pancreas releases insulin, which travels through the blood to regulate how much glucose distant tissues like the liver and muscles absorb.

Juxtacrine Signaling

This happens when cells talk to each other directly. On the outside of one cell, molecules connect to receptors on the outside of another cell. Antigen-presenting cells and T-cells work together in the immune system to start an immune reaction.

Key Players in Cellular Communication

Cells need a few key things to be able to talk to each other properly:

Signaling Molecules

These chemicals enable cells to communicate with each other and transmit messages. Some examples are:

- **Hormones,** like insulin and thyroid hormones, control growth and metabolism.
- **Neurotransmitters,** like serotonin and acetylcholine, make it easier for nerve cells to talk to each other.
- **Cytokines:** They aid in the coordination of the defense system.

- **Growth Factors:** Help cells divide and heal themselves.

Receptors

Receptors are proteins that are inside or on the outside of cells. Certain communication molecules, known as "keys," serve as the "locks" with which they interact. Turning on a receptor initiates a series of events within the cell. Insulin attaches to receptors on fat and muscle cells, telling them to take glucose from the blood.

Second Messengers

When a receptor activates, it frequently sends second messengers, which are tiny molecules inside the cell that enhance the signal. Cyclic AMP (cAMP) is a common second messenger that activates enzymes and other proteins, causing cells to react.

Enzymes and Proteins

Cells communicate through proteins that transmit and receive messages. These proteins can turn on or off processes inside cells, like metabolism or gene production. There are various types of cell signals and their functions.

Types of Cellular Signals and Their Effects

Cells communicate with each other using a variety of message types. Here are some of the primary types of messages and their functions:

Hormonal Signals

In the long run, hormones control things like growth, metabolism, and reproduction. For example, the hormone cortisol helps the body deal with worry by making more energy available.

Electrical Signals

Nerve cells, also known as neurons, quickly send electrical impulses across the body. For muscles to tighten, senses to work, and the brain to work, these impulses are necessary.

Immune Signals

Immune cells send out molecules like cytokines that tell other immune cells to go to the site of the illness or injury. This makes sure that the immune system works together to fight it.

Stress Signals

Stressed cells send out signals to initiate repair processes or, in the worst cases, apoptosis (programmed cell death) to protect neighboring cells from damage.

Cellular Regulation and Homeostasis

Cellular regulation keeps the inside of cells stable while they react to changes in the outside world. Feedback loops maintain this balance, which is crucial for life.

Feedback Mechanisms

Negative Feedback

Negative input is the most common method of controlling systems. Imagine it as a thermostat that halts processes upon reaching the desired outcome.

The pancreas produces insulin when blood sugar levels rise after a meal. Insulin lowers blood sugar. Once we reach normal amounts, insulin production decreases.

Positive Feedback

Positive input doesn't stop a process; it speeds it up. This doesn't happen very often, but it can be helpful sometimes.

During labor, the hormone oxytocin makes the uterus tighten more, which causes the body to release even more oxytocin until the baby is born.

How Dysregulation Leads to Disease

Damaged contact or regulation between cells can result in illness. Here are some ways that an imbalance can negatively impact your health:

Diabetes

In type 2 diabetes, cells stop responding to insulin, which makes it harder for them to take in glucose. This keeps blood sugar levels high all the time.

Cancer

Cancer cells often take over communication pathways, which lets them grow out of control and avoid signals that would usually kill cells.

Autoimmune Disorders

The immune system attacks healthy cells when someone has an autoimmune disease like rheumatoid arthritis.

Neurological Disorders

Diseases like Parkinson's disease, sadness, and anxiety are characterized by imbalanced neurotransmitter signaling.

The Role of Nutrition in Cellular Communication

Nutrition is crucial for helping cells talk to each other and keep things in balance. Lack of some nutrients can damage communication pathways, while too much of others can make them work better. Some important examples are:

- Omega-3 fatty acids: change the creation of cytokines to improve neuronal signaling and lower inflammation.

- Antioxidants, like vitamins C and E, keep cells safe from oxidative stress and make sure that signaling pathways keep working.
- Making ATP, a chemical that powers numerous signaling processes, requires magnesium.
- B vitamins help the body use energy and make hormones like dopamine and serotonin.

How to Support Healthy Cellular Communication

To improve cell phone regulation and conversation, think about the following ideas:

Eat a Balanced Diet

Choose whole foods that are high in vitamins, minerals, and antioxidants.

Stay Hydrated

If properly hydrated, cells can move signaling molecules around.

Exercise Regularly

Being active makes insulin work better, balances neurotransmitters better, and lowers inflammation.

Manage Stress

Chronic stress, especially cortisol, disrupts hormonal messaging and can harm the immune system and metabolism.

Avoid Toxins

Limit your exposure to harmful substances like booze, tobacco, and pesticides that can mess up signaling pathways.

The Impact of Cellular Health on Aging and Disease

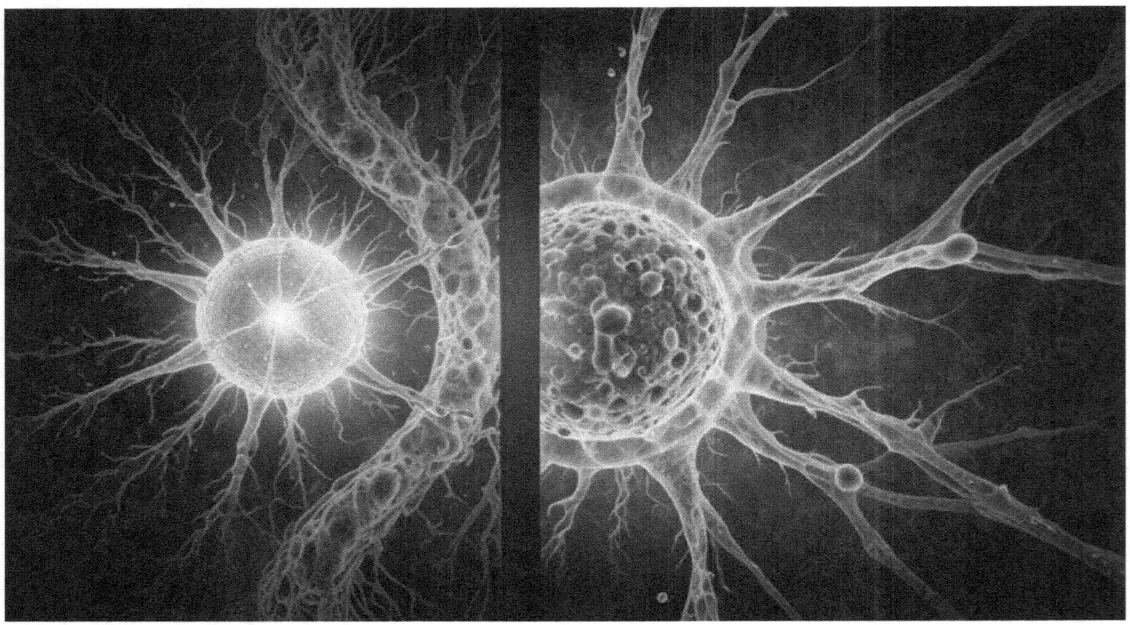

Your general health reflects the health of your cells. When cells are working at their best, the body can fix damage, fight off illness, and stay healthy. But when the health of cells gets worse, the body as a whole feels it.

Aging and Cellular Decline

Cellular performance slowly decreases with age, which is a normal part of life. Some of the main things that cause cells to age are:

Telomere shortening: The caps known as telomeres serve to protect the ends of chromosomes. Telomeres get shorter with each cell division, which causes cells to senesce and finally die.

Malfunctioning mitochondria: As mitochondria age, their ability to produce ATP decreases, leading to fatigue and a slowdown in the aging process of your organs.

Over time, ROS, UV light, and chemicals can cause damage to DNA. Failure to fix this can lead to mutations and cell failure.

Disease and Cellular Dysfunction

Cellular health problems are the cause of many long-term illnesses. As an example:

Cellular insulin communication issues make it difficult for cells to absorb glucose, which leads to diabetes.

Alzheimer's and other neurodegenerative diseases are associated with issues with mitochondria and oxidative stress in brain cells.

Cancer: Changes in DNA and issues with their management cause cells to grow out of control.

The best way to avoid these conditions is to keep your cells healthy through proper nutrition, exercise, and living choices.

Cells are the building blocks of life and the machines that make your body work. We can learn how cells stay healthy and avoid disease by studying their structure, energy production, communication, and health factors. In the next chapters, we'll look at how food, lifestyle, and targeted interventions can improve the health of cells and make the body stronger and healthier.

CHAPTER 2

THE CELLULAR ENERGY EQUATION – WHY IT MATTERS

Life is based on energy. At the level of the cells, every heartbeat, breath, thought, and action depends on a steady flow of energy. Even the most basic things that the body does can't happen without energy. This chapter talks about the complicated processes that make and move energy within cells, as well as the important roles that oxygen, nutrition, and detoxification play. It also talks about how problems with cellular health can cause tiredness, disease, and old age. To find vigor and long-term health, you need to understand the cellular energy equation.

How Energy Flows Through Your Cells

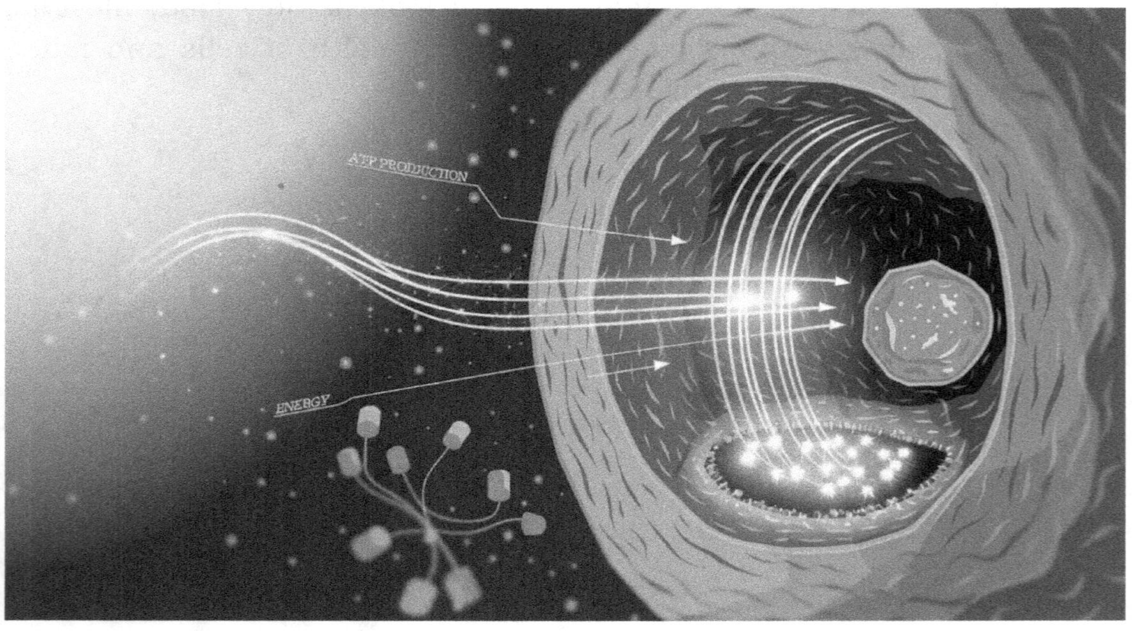

The power of cells to make energy is what makes life possible. All living things need this energy to do their jobs, from DNA repair and immune defense to muscle movement and brain activity. This process of energy flow starts with the food you eat and the air you breathe. The body converts these into adenosine triphosphate (ATP), its "energy currency."

The Basics of Cellular Energy Production

Mitochondria: The Power Plants of the Cell

Almost all cells have mitochondria, which are specific parts of cells. Their primary function is to produce ATP through a process known as cellular   metabolism. Mitochondria are special because they have their own DNA, which lets them change and adapt to meet the body's energy needs. For long-term energy creation, mitochondria must work properly.

ATP: The Energy Currency

The molecule ATP saves energy and sends it to the parts of the cell that need it. When you move a muscle, think a thought, or digest food, your body produces Adenosine diphosphate (ADP), which provides the necessary   energy   for   these   activities. Every second, the body makes and uses billions of ATP molecules, which shows how important it is to make energy efficiently.

The Stages of Cellular Respiration

Cellular respiration is the process by which your cells turn air and food into ATP. There are three main stages:

Glycolysis

Energy production begins in the cell's cytoplasm. The breakdown of glucose (sugar) into two units of pyruvate produces a small amount of ATP.

Although glycolysis doesn't require oxygen, it isn't as efficient as subsequent steps.

The Krebs Cycle (Citric Acid Cycle)

Several chemical reactions further break down pyruvate when it enters the mitochondria. As a result, this process makes carbon dioxide and high-energy electron carriers (NADH and FADH2). The Krebs Cycle is an important step because it gives the next stage of energy production the building blocks it needs.

The Electron Transport Chain (ETC)

The ETC is the last and most efficient step in making energy. It takes place in the mitochondria's inner membrane.

Some proteins pass high-energy electrons from NADH and FADH2 along them. This creates a gradient that propels the synthesis of ATP. As the final electron donor, oxygen plays a crucial role in maintaining the chain's functionality.

This step is crucial for maintaining the energy flow, as it produces the majority of ATP.

The Role of Energy Flow in Daily Life

Every part of life depends on the energy that cellular respiration produces, such as:

Physical Activity: For muscle cells to tighten and move, they need a lot of ATP.

Brain Function: Even though the brain is small, it uses about 20% of the body's energy to do things like think, remember, and concentrate.

Immune Defense: To fight infections, heal wounds, and keep up a strong defense against germs, immune cells need energy.

Blocking energy flow can exhaust you, impair your performance, and weaken your defense system.

The Role of Oxygen, Nutrition, and Detoxification

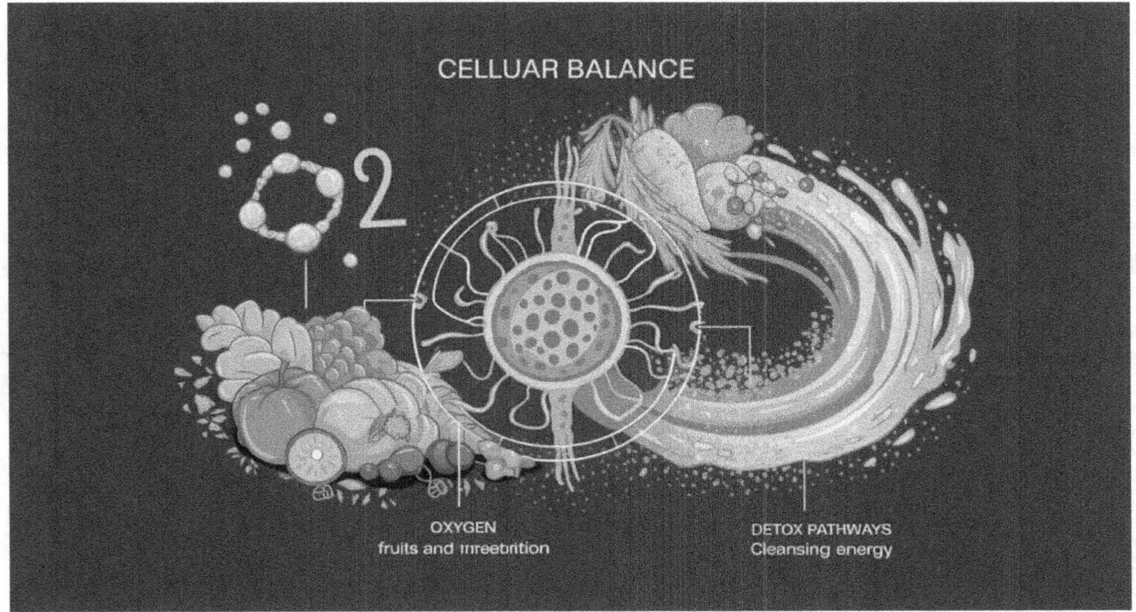

Three important things affect the flow of energy through your cells: air, food, and the ability to get rid of waste. Together, these parts make up the building blocks for cells to work well.

Oxygen: The Breath of Life

Oxygen is necessary for the final stages of cellular respiration to function. ATP creation stops because the electron transport chain can't work without enough oxygen. When there isn't enough oxygen in the blood (hypoxia), cells switch to anaerobic respiration, which is less efficient. It produces lactic acid and significantly less ATP, leading to fatigue and soreness.

How to Support Oxygenation:

Do physical exercise regularly to get more oxygen to your cells.

Do deep breathing exercises to get more air into your body.

Eat foods that are high in iron, folate, and vitamin B12 to keep your red blood cell count healthy. These foods help move oxygen around the body.

Nutrition: Fuel for Energy Production

The food you eat is the first thing that turns into energy. The cellular respiration route breaks down proteins, fats, and carbohydrates into smaller pieces. However, certain foods play a crucial role in facilitating the functioning of mitochondria and the flow of energy.

Macronutrients

Carbohydrates provide glucose, the primary fuel for glycolysis. When you break down fats, you get fatty acids, which are a major source of energy for long periods of time.

When fats and carbohydrates are insufficient, we use proteins as an additional source of energy.

Micronutrients

B vitamins help the body use energy by working as coenzymes. For example, the body needs niacin, a type of vitamin B3, to make NADH.

The enzyme processes that produce ATP require magnesium.

Coenzyme Q10 (CoQ10) is a strong antioxidant that also helps the mitochondria move electrons around.

How to Optimize Nutrition for Energy:

Eat a healthy diet full of whole, unprocessed foods.

Leafy veggies, nuts, seeds, and lean protein are all sources that are high in nutrients.

Stay away from processed foods and too much sugar, as they can damage mitochondria over time.

Detoxification: Clearing Cellular Waste

When cells produce energy, they produce waste products such as carbon dioxide, free radicals, and other toxins. If not properly cleared, these waste products can damage cell structures and stop energy flow.

How to Support Detoxification:

Drink plenty of water to get rid of toxins.

To fight free radicals, eat foods that are high in antioxidants, like dark chocolate and nuts.

Cruciferous veggies, like broccoli and kale, help the liver work better by making detoxification enzymes stronger.

Cellular Stress: What It Is and How It Affects You

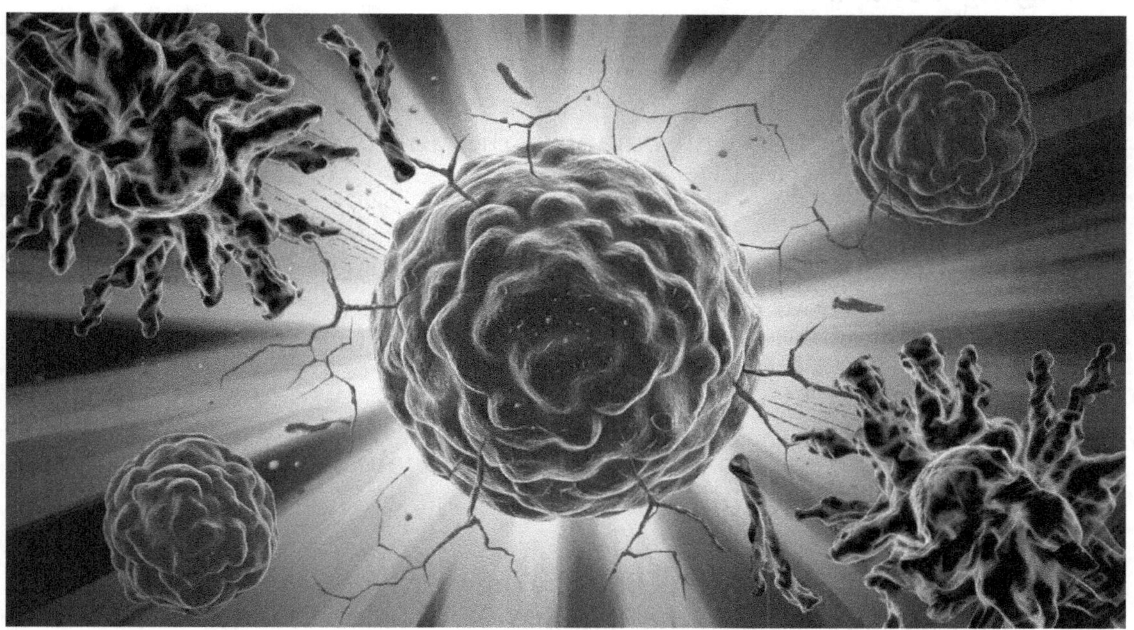

Unrest in cellular stability leads to an imbalance in the internal environment of the cell. This is called cellular stress. Toxins in the environment, inadequate nutrition, not getting enough sleep, and even emotional worry can all cause this stress. Stress can lead to cellular swelling, which can have numerous detrimental effects on the body.

The Impact of Cellular Stress

Cellular stress can have an effect on many body processes, such as:

Energy production: Stressed-out cells may have malfunctioning mitochondria, leading to fatigue and low energy levels.

Inflammation: Cellular stress that lasts for a long time can lead to long-lasting inflammation, which raises the risk of chronic diseases like cancer, diabetes, and heart disease.

Immune system: Weak immune cells can increase the risk of illness.

Skin health: Cellular stress can cause acne, eczema, and other skin problems.

Managing Cellular Stress

To lower cellular stress, pay attention to:

Nutrition: Eat a healthy, well-balanced diet full of fruits, veggies, whole grains, and beneficial fats.

Hydration: Drink a lot of water to help your body get rid of toxins.

Sleep: Aim for 7 to 9 hours of sleep each night to help keep your cells working properly.

Managing your stress: Do things that make you feel better, like yoga, meditation, or deep breathing routines.

Supplements: To help your cells stay healthy, you might want to eat more vitamins and omega-3 fatty acids.

How Poor Cellular Health Leads to Fatigue, Disease, and Aging

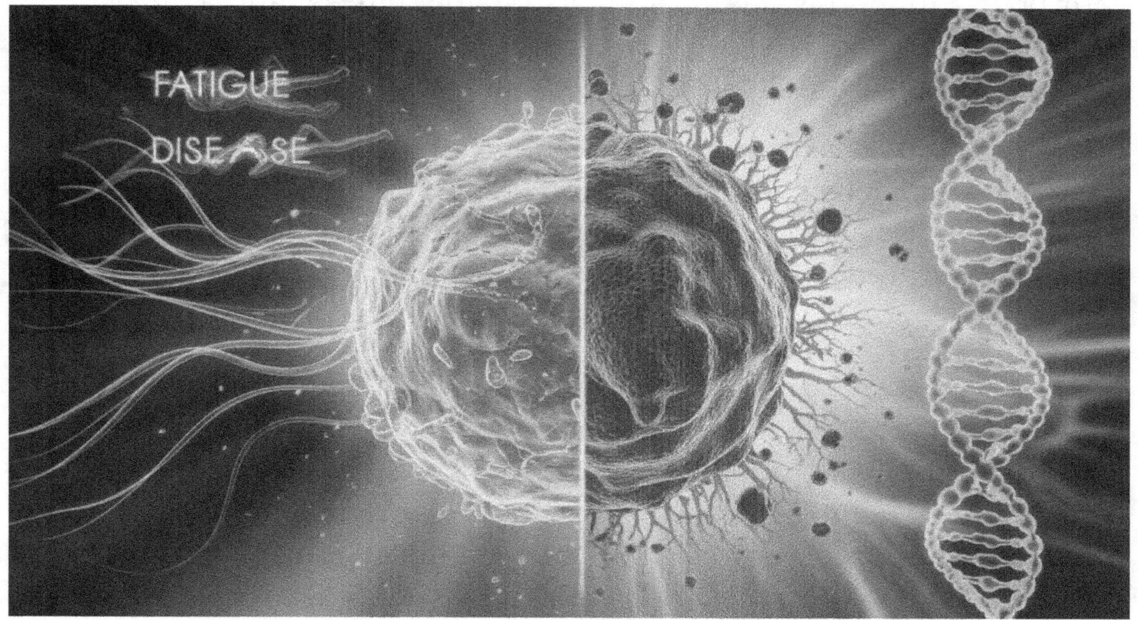

Cellular health is the most important part of general health. As a highly specialized machine, each of the trillions of cells that make up the human body has specific tasks and jobs that are necessary to keep the body alive and well. When the health of cells gets worse, it can set off a chain of adverse events that can cause tiredness, chronic diseases, and faster aging. Figuring out how cellular dysfunction affects these results is important for coming up with healthy eating and living habits that will help you live longer.

1. The Role of Cellular Function in Health

Cells are the building blocks of life. Each cell does many things, such as making energy, taking in nutrients, getting rid of trash, talking to each other, and fixing things. Adenosine triphosphate (ATP) is the main source of energy for most cells. Cellular respiration in the mitochondria, sometimes referred to as the "powerhouses" of the cell, produces it.

A healthy cell can do its job well, helping the body's processes and protecting itself from things that could be stressful. Conversely, unhealthy cells disrupt these processes. This leads to a worsening of your body's functions, manifesting as fatigue, illness, and aging.

2. The Cellular Energy Crisis: Fatigue as a Primary Symptom

Being fatigued is a common sign that your cells are not healthy. It happens when cells can't make enough energy to meet the needs of the body. The mitochondria are crucial to this process, and if they aren't working right, the body may not have enough energy.

Mitochondrial Dysfunction

Mitochondria can malfunction due to genetic changes, toxic stress, poor diet, insufficient exercise, or exposure to toxins. Damage to mitochondria reduces their efficiency in producing ATP, thereby reducing the cell's energy source. This can make you feel slow, tired all the time, and unable to handle things. Not only do the muscles feel weak, but so do the brain cells, immune cells, and organs. This can cause mental tiredness and trouble focusing.

Oxidative Stress and Free Radical Damage

In order to make energy, cells automatically make reactive oxygen species (ROS). Cell communication and the immune system depend on ROS, yet an excess of them can harm proteins, lipids, and DNA in cells, a condition known as oxidative stress. This damage makes cells less effective and speeds up the aging process, which can lead to chronic tiredness. Foods that contain antioxidants, like flavonoids, vitamin C, and vitamin E, help fight these free radicals and keep cells working well.

3. Inflammation and Immune System Disruption

"Inflammaging," also known as chronic low-grade inflammation, indicates unhealthy cells and is associated with both illness and aging. Over time, excessive or chronic inflammation can harm tissues and organs, despite the body's inflammatory response protecting against damage and infection.

Cellular Inflammation

Oxidative stress, inadequate nutrition, and exposure to environmental toxins are some of the things that can cause inflammation at the cellular level. Cytokines are messaging molecules that immune cells, especially macrophages and white blood cells, release. These molecules make inflammation worse. Damage to cellular structures can happen over time due to chronic inflammation. This reduces the effectiveness of cells, leading to fatigue and exacerbating the effects of chronic diseases.

Autoimmune Disorders

Autoimmune diseases such as lupus, rheumatoid arthritis, and multiple sclerosis occur when the immune system begins to attack healthy cells. Not only are these situations painful, but they can also hurt the health and function of cells, making fatigue worse and raising the risk of getting another disease.

4. The Link Between Poor Cellular Health and Disease

A lack of healthy cells is a cause of many long-term illnesses, ranging from heart diseases and cancer to neurological diseases. Typically, a combination of mitochondrial dysfunction, oxidative damage, and long-term inflammation characterizes these situations.

Cardiovascular Disease

Your heart and blood passageways depend on the health of the cells that line them. These cells are called endothelial cells. Damage to endothelial cells can cause atherosclerosis (artery hardening and narrowing), high blood pressure, and heart problems. High LDL cholesterol and high blood sugar exacerbate this damage by inducing inflammation and reactive stress.

Cancer

Changes in genes often cause cells to multiply and grow out of control, leading to cancer. Cells in poor health are more susceptible to mutations that can lead to cancerous changes due to DNA damage and malfunctioning healing systems. Lifestyle choices like inadequate nutrition, smoking, and long-term worry can speed up this process by making cells more vulnerable to damage and making it harder for them to repair it.

Neurodegenerative Diseases

Cells, especially neurons, lose their ability to work properly in Alzheimer's disease, Parkinson's disease, and other neurological diseases. Brain inflammation and problems with mitochondria can kill cells and make it harder to think and remember things. Over time, oxidative stress can cause abnormal protein deposits to build up, which can hurt brain cells even more.

5. Aging and Cellular Health: The Accelerated Decline

Aging and cell health are inseparable. Because oxidative stress, DNA mutations, and cellular aging all do damage over time, cells slowly lose their ability to do their job.

Cellular Senescence

When cells reach cellular senescence, they can no longer grow or work properly. Senescent cells often give off chemicals that are harmful for the body and can hurt nearby tissues and cause inflammation. Over time, these cells build up and make tissues less functional. This exacerbates aging signs such as less flexible skin and organ dysfunction.

Telomere Shortening

Cells split many times a day, and each time, the protective caps on the ends of chromosomes get shorter. Once the telomeres become too short, cells are unable to grow. Senescent cells die at this point. This process limits the ability of tissues and systems to grow back, which causes physical and mental abilities to decline with age.

Reduced Autophagy

Autophagy is the process by which cells get rid of broken parts and reuse them to keep the cell healthy. When we get older, autophagy works less well, which causes broken-down cell parts to build up. This increases your susceptibility to age-related diseases and accelerates the breakdown of body parts.

6. Strategies to Support Cellular Health

The positive news is that targeted changes to diet and lifestyle can improve many areas of cellular health. Supporting the health of cells can help lower the risk of getting sick, feeling tired, and aging faster than you should.

Diet and Nutrition

Foods rich in antioxidants, healthy fats, and essential vitamins and minerals can protect cells from harm. Foods like berries, leafy greens, nuts, seeds, and fatty fish contain many substances that help mitochondria stay healthy and lower oxidative stress.

Exercise

Regular exercise improves the health of cells by increasing the function of mitochondria and encouraging autophagy. Studies have demonstrated that strength training and aerobic exercise enhance the quantity of mitochondria in cells. This makes it easier for cells to make energy and fix themselves.

Sleep and Stress Management

Getting enough adequate sleep and lowering your stress levels are also important for fixing cells and making energy. Sleep can repair cellular processes, but prolonged worry can exacerbate inflammation and oxidative damage. Mindfulness, meditation, and deep breathing are some of the techniques that can help you deal with stress and keep your cells healthy in general.

Not having healthy cells isn't just a result of getting older; it's also a major cause of fatigue, illness, and the aging process itself. Understanding how cellular dysfunction happens and how it affects the body helps us understand how important it is to keep cells healthy through food, exercise, and lifestyle choices. A healthier life starts with healthy cells, and by making sure cells work at their best, we can avoid getting sick and live a longer, healthier life.

In the upcoming chapters, we will discuss specific dietary and lifestyle changes that can maintain the health of your cells and combat the factors that lead to fatigue, illness, and aging.

CHAPTER 3

CELLULAR HEALTH AND LONGEVITY – THE CONNECTION

There are a lot of people who want to live a long life, but not just any old life. People want to live a long, healthy, and full life. At the heart of this goal is the health of our cells, which has a huge impact on both the length and quality of our lives. The link between healthy cells and living a long time is complicated and multifaceted. It involves complex biological processes that manage growth, repair, and the aging process itself. This section delves into the science of cellular health, examining the impact of telomeres, cellular repair, and the aging process on cells. It also shows how improving the function of cells can help people live longer and healthier lives.

The Science behind Longevity and Cellular Health

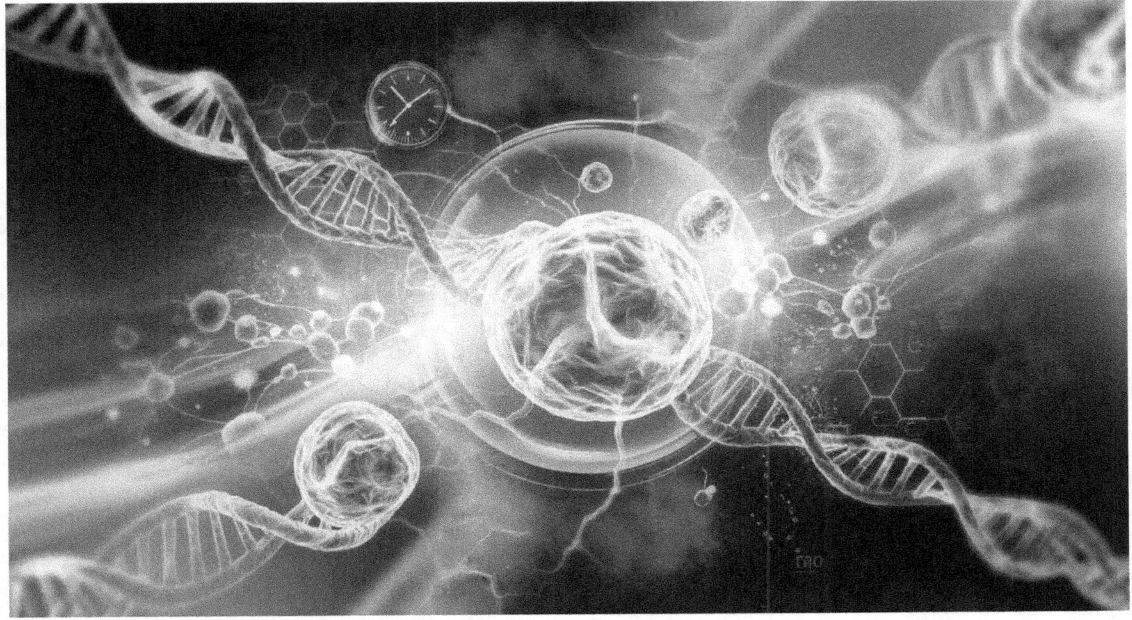

People who try to live longer don't just want to live longer; they want to live a life full of energy, health, and few illnesses. The science of living a long life closely correlates with the health of our cells, which serve as the foundation of life and regulate nearly all bodily functions. The things that control the health of cells, like how they make energy, fix themselves, and react to stress, have a direct effect on how long and how well we live. This section will delve into the scientific underpinnings of why healthy cells contribute to longer lifespans. It will demonstrate how various cellular processes contribute to aging and provide strategies for maintaining long-term health.

Cellular Aging and Its Impact on the Body

Cellular aging is the slow process by which cells lose their ability to work and stay together over time. This makes us older and more likely to get sick. Cellular damage and repair—or their balance—drive aging. Cellular health goes down when damage is greater than repair, which adds to the physical and functional decline that comes with getting older.

Cellular Damage and Stress

Damage to cells caused by oxidative stress is one of the main ways that cells age. Cells produce unstable molecules known as free radicals during regular activities. They can react with DNA, proteins, and lipids in cells, damaging their structure. Such damage can alter the DNA, reducing the usefulness of the cell and eventually leading to age-related   diseases.
To protect itself from oxidative stress, the body has antioxidant enzymes (like superoxide dismutase and catalase) and antioxidants that come from food (like vitamins C and E). The body's antioxidant protections, on the other hand, get weaker with age, which lets oxidative damage build up.

Mitochondrial Decline

The "powerhouses" of the cell, mitochondria, produce energy through a process known as cellular respiration. Over time, oxidative stress, genetic mutations, and other factors can damage mitochondria, reducing their ability to produce energy. This loss of mitochondrial function can make you tired, weak in muscles, unable to think clearly, and less able to fix and maintain tissues. Problems with mitochondria often link to age-related diseases like Alzheimer's, Parkinson's, and heart disease.

DNA Damage and Mutations

Things like UV rays, pollution, and metabolic byproducts constantly damage the DNA in our cells. There are ways for cells to fix DNA damage, but as cells age, these ways work less well. DNA damage and mutations that build up over time can make cells less effective and help age-related diseases like cancer grow.

Telomere Shortening

Telomeres, which are caps that protect the ends of chromosomes, are a key way to tell how old a cell is. Telomeres get shorter every time a cell splits. Telomeres play a crucial role in maintaining the stability of the genetic code and preventing damage to the ends of chromosomes. When telomeres get too short, the cell either goes into senescence, a biologically active state where it doesn't divide, or it dies through apoptosis. Shorter telomeres contribute to cells' reduced ability to heal and increased susceptibility to age-related diseases.

Telomeres, Cellular Repair, and the Aging Process

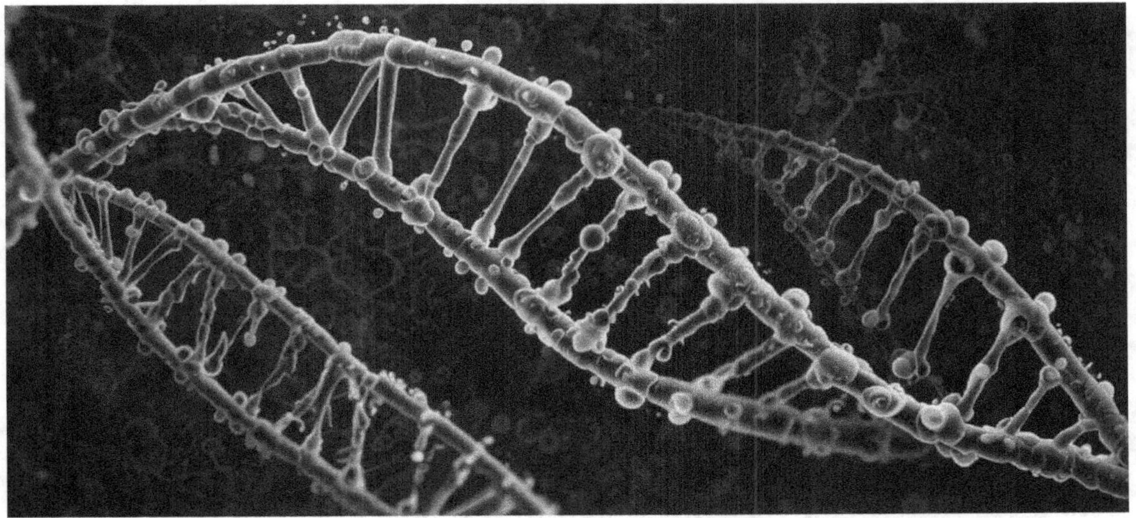

Telomeres are essential parts of knowing how cells stay healthy and live a long time. These DNA patterns that repeat at the ends of chromosomes keep the genetic material safe while the cell divides. Telomeres get shorter every time a cell splits, which makes it harder for the cell to replicate and work properly over time.

The Role of Telomeres

The protected caps on shoelaces are like telomeres. They keep the ends of chromosomes from fraying and sticking to each other. As cells divide, telomeres get shorter. This instructs the cell to either cease its division or undergo a controlled cell death process known as apoptosis. This normal process helps stop old or damaged cells from multiplying and possibly turning into cancer.

However, aging-related diseases and conditions such as heart disease, diabetes, and neurodegenerative illnesses are also associated with telomere shortening. Numerous factors, including genes, food, stress, and lifestyle choices, can alter the rate of telomere shortening.

Telomere Length as a Marker of Aging

You can use telomere length to determine a cell's age. Even if a person is young in years, shorter telomeres show that they are biologically older. Bad eating habits, long-term worry, not getting enough sleep, and smoking can all shorten telomeres faster. Conversely, studies have demonstrated that regular exercise, a healthy diet rich in antioxidants, and effective stress management can prolong telomeres and enhance cell life.

Telomerase and Cellular Repair

By adding repeating DNA sequences, an enzyme known as telomerase can lengthen telomeres. This enzyme, which stem cells and some defense cells use, helps them maintain their ability to grow new cells. Most cells, though, don't have much telomerase activity, and cells lose the ability to fix and renew themselves as their telomeres get shorter. Scientists have been very interested in the idea of activating or adding to telomerase because it might make cells live longer and delay the start of aging and diseases related to getting older. However, unintentionally activating telomerase carries risks, including an increased risk of developing cancer.

How Optimizing Cellular Function Can Add Years to Your Life

Getting cells to work at their best is key to living longer and having a satisfactory quality of life. People can support the health of their cells and lengthen their lives in a number of ways, including:

Balanced Nutrition and Antioxidants

Eating a lot of vitamins can help fight off free radicals and oxidative stress. Foods like nuts, seeds, fruits, and veggies are full of antioxidants and important minerals and vitamins that keep cells healthy. People who follow a Mediterranean diet are more likely to live longer and be less likely to get age-related diseases. This diet includes lots of fruits and veggies, healthy fats (like olive oil), and whole grains.

Caloric Restriction and Intermittent Fasting

Animal models have shown that calorie restriction, which means eating fewer calories without becoming malnourished, can make people live longer. This method seems to improve the body's ability to deal with stress, speed up autophagy, and make mitochondria work better. The benefits of intermittent fasting are similar, but it involves not eating for extended periods of time. Intermittent fasting can help cells stay healthy and may even make people live longer by encouraging autophagy and cellular repair.

Regular Physical Activity

Working out is one of the best things for cell health. It speeds up the repair of cells and increases mitochondrial biogenesis, which is the process of making new mitochondria. Regular exercise can reduce reactive stress, enhance blood flow, safeguard the heart, and maintain a healthy length of telomeres. It also helps your brain work better and lowers your risk of getting chronic diseases.

Adequate Sleep

In order for cells to repair and heal, it is essential that you get enough quality sleep. While you sleep, your body performs processes that aid in the proper functioning of cells and the repair of damage. Not getting enough or adequate sleep can speed up aging and make it harder for the body to deal with stress and heal from injuries. Keeping a regular sleep routine and making sure your bedroom is dark and quiet are examples of excellent sleep hygiene that can help you sleep better and live longer.

Dealing with Stress

Stress that lasts for a long time can damage cells and speed up the aging process. Worry activates the hypothalamic-pituitary-adrenal (HPA) axis, leading to the production of more stress hormones such as cortisol. High amounts of cortisol can make inflammation worse, weaken the immune system, and lead to oxidative damage. Meditation, yoga, deep breathing, and being mindful are all stress management methods that can help lower stress and improve the health of cells.

Supplements and Natural Compounds

Researchers have looked into some supplements and chemicals to see if they can help cells stay healthy and live longer. Some of these are:

- As an example, coenzyme Q10 (CoQ10) helps mitochondria work and makes energy.
- Resveratrol: Red wine and certain plants contain this chemical. Studies have demonstrated that it activates sirtuins, proteins responsible for regulating cell repair and longevity.
- Curcumin is the main ingredient in turmeric. It is known to reduce inflammation and protect cells from damage.

- Components of NAD+: Nicotinamide riboside contributes to the synthesis of NAD+, a molecule essential for DNA repair and energy processing in cells.

The study of living a long life is complicated and encompasses many areas. However, the health of our cells is at the core of this field. Numerous factors contribute to aging, such as cell damage, inefficient healing, and issues with mitochondrial function. Nevertheless, if we understand how cells age and take steps to improve their function, we might be able to live longer and enjoy the years we have left better. Eating right, working out, getting enough sleep, dealing with stress, and taking specific supplements can all help keep cells healthy and extend life. By using these tips, we can help our bodies naturally heal and regenerate, which will eventually help us live longer and healthier lives.

PART 2:

OPTIMIZING CELLULAR HEALTH THROUGH DIET

CHAPTER 4

THE ROLE OF NUTRITION IN CELLULAR ENERGY

Every cell in your body functions like a busy machine, continuously producing the energy your brain, muscles, and organs require through a process known as cellular respiration. Nutrition plays a crucial role in this process by providing the raw materials cells need to produce energy.

Important nutrients like glucose from carbohydrates, fatty acids from good fats, and amino acids from proteins break down into adenosine triphosphate (ATP), the cell's main source of energy. In addition to these macronutrients, micronutrients like iron, magnesium, B vitamins, and copper are crucial because they work with enzymes to produce energy.

Not getting enough nutrients can mess up this complicated process, making you tired, slowing down cell repair, and weakening your defense system. For the best energy for cells, you should focus on nutrient-dense foods that give you steady energy without making your blood sugar levels go up and down.

Energy is what makes life possible, and the body gets its energy from cells, which are the smallest functional unit. A very well-tuned system inside each cell works nonstop to turn the food you eat into adenosine triphosphate (ATP), which is a form of energy that your body can use. Knowing how this process works helps you understand why nutrition is essential for making energy in cells and for your health in general.

The Energy Production Process: Cellular Respiration

Cells use cellular respiration to turn the nutrients they get from food into ATP. Cellular respiration involves several steps, each of which requires a distinct set of nutrients for optimal functioning:

Glycolysis:

Cells break down glucose, which comes from carbohydrates, in the first step, known as glycolysis, to produce a small amount of ATP.

Key Nutrients: The main things that give us glucose are complex carbohydrates, like whole grains and starchy veggies.

Krebs Cycle (Citric Acid Cycle):

This is where the products from glycolysis enter the mitochondria. Here, nutrients are broken down even more, and NADH and FADH2 are made, which are high-energy molecules.

Some important nutrients are vitamins B1 (thiamine), B2 (riboflavin), B3 (niacin), and B5 (pantothenic acid). They work with other nutrients in this cycle as coenzymes.

Electron Transport Chain: Most of ATP is made from the molecules with a lot of energy that were made earlier. Oxygen is crucial because it takes in the last electron.

Key Nutrients: Hemoglobin contains iron, which helps oxygen get to where it needs to go. Copper and coenzyme Q10 help move electrons around.

Macronutrients: The Building Blocks of Energy

Carbohydrates, proteins, and fats are the three macronutrients. They all play different roles in making energy:

Carbohydrates:

Carbohydrates give the body energy, especially when doing tasks that require a lot of it. Glucose is quickly turned into ATP from glucose, which comes from carbohydrates.

Quinoa, brown rice, oats, sweet potatoes, and fruits like apples and bananas are the best places to get it.

Fats*:*

As an energy source, fats burn more slowly but for a longer duration. In the mitochondria, a process known as beta-oxidation breaks down fatty acids.

Avocados, nuts, fatty fish (like salmon), and olive oil are the best places to get it.

Proteins*:*

The body primarily uses proteins to repair and maintain cells, but it can also convert amino acids into glucose when it doesn't have enough energy.

Eggs, soy, beans, lentils, and lean meat are the best sources.

Micronutrients: The Hidden Heroes

However, micronutrients are not direct energy sources because they are required for the enzyme processes that produce ATP.

B vitamins, like B1, B2, B3, B5, and B6, help turn carbs, proteins, and fats into energy that the body can use.

Whole grains, cheese, meat, leafy greens, and cereals with added vitamins and minerals are all good sources.

Magnesium*:*

ATP is made with the help of magnesium, which also helps keep the shape of ATP molecules stable.

Leafy greens, nuts, dark chocolate, and black beans are all sources.

Iron*:*

Helps oxygen get to cells through hemoglobin, making sure cells have enough oxygen to make energy.

Red meat, lentils, spinach, and grains with added vitamins and minerals are good sources.

Coenzyme Q10 (CoQ10):

The mitochondria need it to move electrons around. Chronic tiredness can be caused by a deficiency.

Full-fat fish, organ meats, and whole grains are all good sources.

The Role of Oxygen in Cellular Energy

For the last step of making ATP, oxygen is essential. Without oxygen, cells must resort to anaerobic respiration, resulting in reduced energy production and the accumulation of lactic acid, which can lead to cell damage. This is why eating a lot of iron-rich foods and making sure your heart stays healthy by working out regularly are essential for keeping oxygen flowing to cells.

The Impact of Poor Nutrition on Cellular Energy

When you don't eat enough of the right nutrients;

- You may feel fatigued all the time because your body is having trouble making enough ATP.
- ***Mitochondrial Dysfunction: Lack*** of nutrients makes mitochondria less efficient, which lowers energy production and raises the production of free radicals.
- ***Slower Recovery:*** Cells can't fix or grow back properly without enough protein and micronutrients.

Practical Tips for Supporting Cellular Energy

Balance Your Plate:

At every meal, eat a mix of carbs, proteins, and good fats. One meal that has all three macronutrients and important vitamins is grilled salmon, quinoa, and sautéed spinach.

Incorporate Energy-Boosting Snacks:

Pick something like a handful of nuts, an egg that has been hard-boiled, or fruit with nut butter on it.

Stay Hydrated:

Being dehydrated slows down the flow of blood and oxygen to cells, which makes it harder for them to make energy. Drink at least 8 cups of water every day.

Eat Foods That Are High In Iron And Vitamin C:

To improve iron intake, eat foods that are high in vitamin C (like oranges) along with foods that are high in iron (like spinach).

Cut Down On Processed Foods:

Too much sugar and processed carbs can make your energy go up and down, and trans fats may make it harder for your mitochondria to work. If you know how important nutrition is for cellular energy, you can choose foods that give you more energy, make your cells healthier, and support your general health.

What to Eat for Optimal Cellular Function

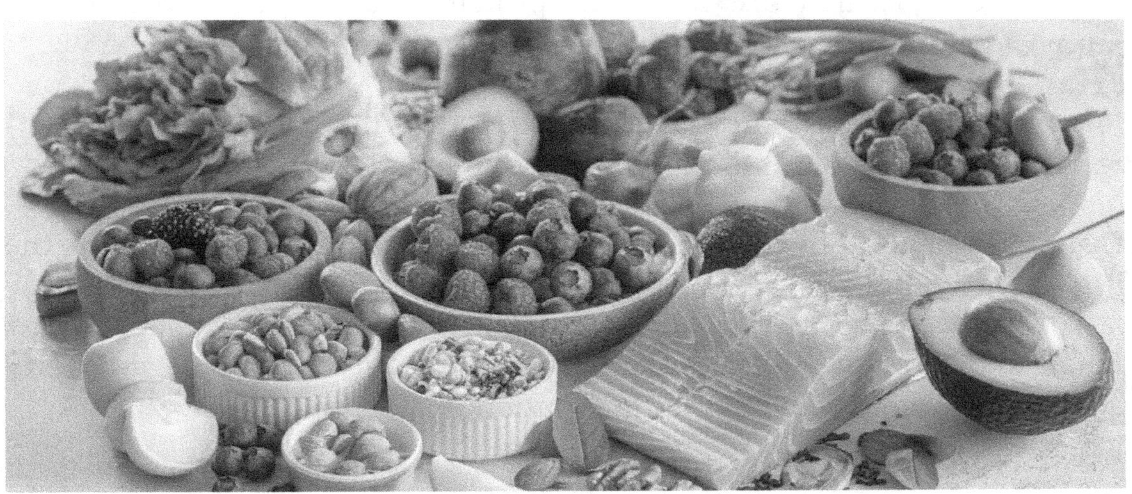

For cells to work properly, they need a steady flow of nutrients that help them make energy, fix themselves, and keep their structure. For this to happen, you need to eat a range of whole foods as part of a balanced diet. It is important to choose foods that are high in nutrients because each group has its own benefits for cell health.

1. Groups of Nutrients For Cellular Optimization

Complex Carbohydrates

Carbohydrates are the main source of energy for cells. Complex carbs, on the other hand, release glucose slowly over time, so blood sugar doesn't go up and down too quickly, which can affect cell energy.

Steady energy for cellular respiration and ATP production is beneficial for cell function.

Quinoa is full of protein and fiber, which gives you energy that lasts.

Sweet potatoes have a lot of beta-carotene and vitamin C, which help protect cells.

Whole grains like brown rice, oats, and barley give cells power that lasts for a long time.

Lean Proteins

Amino acids, which are found in proteins, are used to repair and support cellular structures like DNA, enzymes, and membranes.

It enhances the efficiency of cells by simplifying the process of self-repairing, hormone production, and enzyme activity.

Eggs: They contain choline, which is necessary to maintain the integrity of cell membranes.

Fish: Mackerel and salmon are excellent sources of omega-3 fatty acids, which help cells fight inflammation.

Plant-based options: For vegans, lentils, chickpeas, and tofu are all excellent choices.

Healthy Fats

Fats are essential for keeping cell membranes fluid and permeable, which lets cells share nutrients and waste easily.

Benefits for Cellular Function: helps keep cell membranes healthy and gives cells an extra source of energy.

It is high in vitamin E and monounsaturated fats, which protect cells from toxic stress.

Nuts and seeds: Flaxseeds, almonds, and chia seeds are beneficial sources of antioxidants and important fatty acids.

Olive oil is full of antioxidants and monounsaturated fats, which help cells live longer.

2. Micronutrient Powerhouses for Cellular Function

Micronutrients are important for many biological processes that keep cells healthy. Lack of these nutrients can lead to improper cell function and fatigue.

Antioxidants

Free radical damage reduces oxidative stress, which can reduce the effectiveness of cells.

- Berries: Blueberries, strawberries, and raspberries are rich in flavonoids and vitamin C.
- Dark leafy greens: Spinach and kale are full of lutein and zeaxanthin.
- Green tea has catechins in it, which are strong antioxidants that get rid of free radicals.

Minerals

They are essential for enzyme activities and for maintaining the strength of cell structures.

Magnesium: It aids in the production of ATP and the maintenance of muscle function.
Dark chocolate, spinach, and pumpkin seeds are all rich sources.

Zinc aids in cell healing and maintains a robust defense system. It's present in fruits, nuts, and whole foods.

Iron: Aids cells in absorbing oxygen, thereby enhancing their energy production efficiency.

They incorporate it into red meat, lentils, and grains.

Vitamins

Vitamins enable cells to perform essential functions such as synthesising DNA, repairing damaged cells, and utilizing energy.

Vitamin A helps cells grow and protects the nervous system. It is present in beef, sweet potatoes, and liver.

Vitamin C is important for making collagen and protects cells from damage.
You can find it in oranges, bell peppers, and kiwis.

Energy production and DNA repair require B vitamins like B1, B2, B3, B6, and B12.

You can find it in meat, dairy, and whole carbohydrates.

3. Gut-Healthy Foods for Cellular Efficiency

A healthy gut is necessary for absorbing nutrients, which has a direct effect on the health of cells. Probiotics and prebiotics make the gut microbiome better, which makes it easier for the body to absorb and use nutrition.

Yogurt is full of probiotics, which are beneficial for gut health.

Fermented foods, like kimchi and cabbage, help your body absorb nutrients better.

Asparagus and bananas are prebiotic foods, which means they feed beneficial bacteria in the gut.

4. Hydration and Cellular Function

Cells often overlook the importance of water. It helps move nutrients around, get rid of waste, and speed up chemical reactions inside cells. Even mild dehydration can slow down these processes.

Tips for Optimal Hydration:

Drink 8–10 cups of water every day, or more if you're active or in a hot place.

Eat foods that will keep you hydrated, like oranges, tomatoes, and cucumbers.

5. Foods to Avoid for Cellular Health

Some foods are detrimental for cells because they cause inflammation, oxidative stress, or a lack of nutrients.

Refined sugars cause blood sugar levels to rise quickly, stressing out cells.

Trans fats: Found in processed foods, they reduce the flexibility of cell membranes.

Drinking too much alcohol depletes nutrients like B vitamins and makes mitochondrial function worse.

Daily Meal Plan for Optimal Cellular Function

Breakfast

- *Oatmeal made with whole grains and fresh blueberries, nuts, and honey on top.*
- *A cup of green tea.*

Lunch

- *Grilled salmon salad with spinach, kale, avocado, cherry tomatoes, and olive oil dressing.*

- *A slice of whole-grain bread.*

Snack

- *Greek yogurt with chia seeds and sliced banana.*

Dinner

- *Roasted sweet potatoes, steamed broccoli, and baked chicken breast.*

- *A small piece of dark chocolate (70% cocoa or higher) for dessert.*

Staying Hydrated:

- Drink water with cucumber or lemon added to it throughout the day.

For your cells to work at their best, you should eat a range of foods that are balanced and consistent. Adding these nutrient-dense foods to your diet not only helps keep your cells healthy, but it also gives you more energy, boosts your immune system, and makes you live longer.

The Importance of Micronutrients and Macronutrients

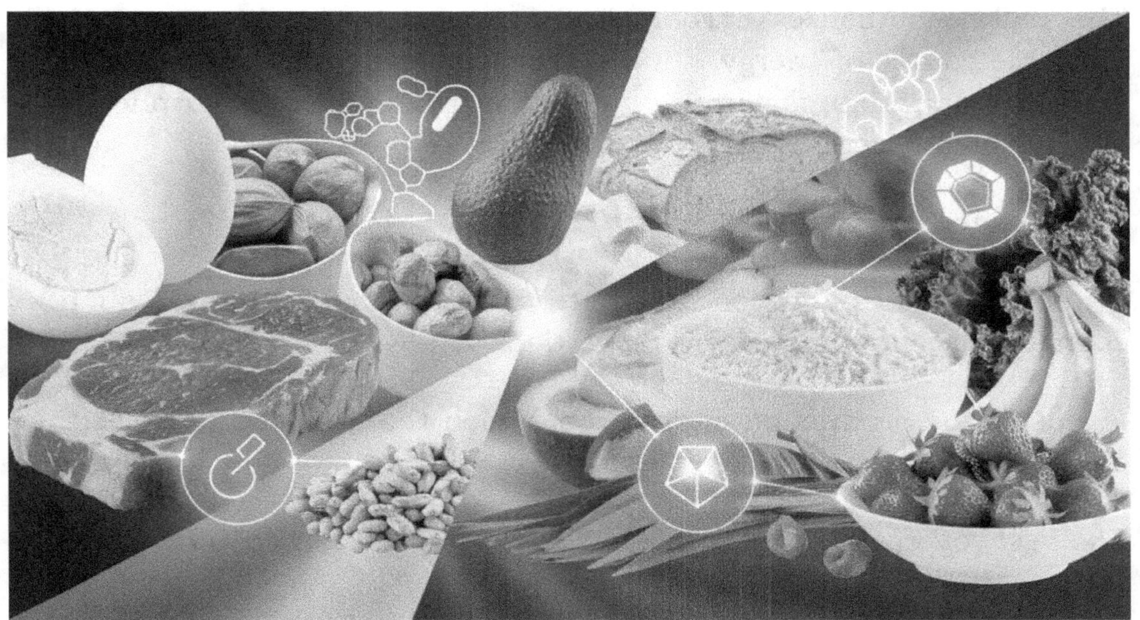

To maintain existence, our bodies depend on two classifications of nutrients: macronutrients, which are required in substantial quantities, and micronutrients, which are necessary in lesser amounts. Collectively, they constitute the cornerstone of cellular health, facilitating energy production, cellular repair, and overall functionality. In the absence of an appropriate equilibrium of these nutrients, cellular functions may deteriorate, resulting in fatigue, compromised immunity, and potential long-term health complications. Let us explore in greater depth the significance of each group.

Macronutrients: The Building Blocks of Cellular Health

Macronutrients are essential nutrients that the body necessitates in substantial quantities for energy production, structural integrity, and biochemical processes. The three principal macronutrients are carbohydrates, proteins, and lipids, each fulfilling distinct and vital functions in cellular activity.

1. Carbohydrates: The Primary Energy Source

The body metabolizes carbohydrates into glucose, the most readily available source of energy. Glucose serves as the primary substrate for cellular respiration, facilitating the synthesis of adenosine triphosphate (ATP), which functions as the energy currency of the cell.

Importance for Cellular Health:

Supplies rapid energy for processes with elevated demands, such as cognitive function and physical exertion.

It aids in the production of glycogen, which the liver and muscles then store for future energy use.

The best sources are whole grains like quinoa, brown rice, and oatmeal.

Fruits, including apples, avocados, and berries.

Sweet potatoes, carrots, and squash are among the vegetables.

2. Proteins: The Repair Crew

Amino acids, which make up proteins, are essential for the synthesis and repair of cellular components like enzymes, membranes, and deoxyribonucleic acid (DNA).

Importance for Cellular Health:

Amino acids play a crucial role in the synthesis of enzymes that enable various cellular processes.

Structural proteins uphold the integrity of cellular membranes and organelles.

Proteins such as hemoglobin facilitate the transport of oxygen, an essential element for the synthesis of adenosine triphosphate (ATP).

Animal-derived: Eggs, lean meats, and fish.

Plant-based sources include lentils, legumes, tofu, and quinoa.

3. Fats: The Protectors and Sustainers

Fats serve not only as a concentrated source of energy but are also essential for maintaining cellular health. They contribute to the formation of the lipid bilayer of cellular membranes, thereby assuring fluidity and safeguarding the contents of the cell.

Importance for Cellular Health:

Omega-3 fatty acids mitigate inflammation, thereby improving cellular function and preventing the onset of chronic diseases.

Adipose tissue serves as a reservoir of energy during periods of deprivation or extended physical exertion.

Fats facilitate the assimilation of fat-soluble vitamins (A, D, E, and K), which are essential for various cellular processes.

The best sources are avocados, almonds, and seeds.

Salmon and sardines are examples of fatty fish.

Use nourishing oils like olive and flaxseed oil.

Micronutrients: The Silent Powerhouses

Micronutrients, encompassing vitamins and minerals, are required in lesser quantities; however, their significance remains undiminished. They function as mediators for enzymatic reactions, serve as structural components, and provide protective mechanisms against oxidative damage.

1. Vitamins: Coenzymes and Cellular Protectors

Vitamins facilitate essential biochemical reactions and safeguard cells from injury induced by free radicals.

Key Vitamins and Their Functions:

- **Vitamin A:** Facilitates cellular differentiation and enhances immune function.
  This is present in carrots, sweet potatoes, and liver.
- **Vitamin C** functions as an antioxidant and facilitates collagen synthesis, thereby contributing to tissue repair.
  It is present in citrus fruits, bell peppers, and asparagus.
- **B Vitamins** (B1, B2, B3, B5, B6, B12) are essential for energy metabolism, DNA synthesis, and the formation of red blood cells.
  It is present in whole grains, dairy products, eggs, and fortified cereals.
- **Vitamin D:** Regulates calcium concentrations, thereby facilitating cellular signaling and promoting skeletal health.
  This can be found in fatty fish, fortified dairy products, and exposure to sunlight.
- **Vitamin E** serves to safeguard cell membranes against oxidative injury.
  Present in: Nuts, seeds, and spinach.

2. Minerals: Structural and Functional Necessities

Minerals are indispensable for both structural components, such as bones, and functional processes, including enzymatic activity.

Key Vitamins and Their Functions:

- **Calcium** is crucial for cellular signaling and the contraction of muscle fibers.
  They are present in dairy products, verdant vegetables, and almonds.
- **Iron:** Essential for the transportation of oxygen to cells and the production of adenosine triphosphate (ATP).
  This is present in red meat, lentils, and fortified cereals.
- **Magnesium** facilitates more than 300 enzymatic reactions, including those involved in the production of adenosine triphosphate (ATP).

This dish is presented with spinach, pumpkin seeds, and dark chocolate.
- ***Zinc:*** Promotes cellular repair and enhances immune function. This is present in shellfish, legumes, and whole grains.
- ***Selenium*** serves as an antioxidant, safeguarding cells from oxidative stress. Brazil nuts, eggs, and tuna are present.

The Symbiotic Relationship between Macronutrients and Micronutrients

Macronutrients and micronutrients function synergistically to uphold optimal cellular performance.

Energy Production:

Macronutrients serve as essential substrates (e.g., glucose, fatty acids) for the generation of energy.

Micronutrients such as magnesium, B vitamins, and iron function as essential cofactors for the enzymes that facilitate the catabolism of these macronutrients.

Cellular Repair and Maintenance:

Proteins supply amino acids essential for the repair process, whereas vitamins such as A and C facilitate the healing process.

Minerals such as zinc and selenium serve to safeguard against injury and facilitate regeneration.

Antioxidant Defense:

Omega-3 fatty acids possess anti-inflammatory properties, while antioxidants such as vitamins C and E, along with selenium, serve to neutralize detrimental free radicals.

Practical Ways to Ensure a Balanced Intake

Enhance Your Dietary Variety:

Integrate an assortment of vibrant fruits and vegetables to ensure a comprehensive intake of essential vitamins and minerals.

Macronutrient Balance:

Strive for a plate composition that consists of 50% vegetables, 25% lean protein, and 25% whole carbohydrates or healthy fats.

Select Whole Foods:

Reduce the consumption of processed foods, as they are frequently devoid of vital micronutrients and may contain detrimental fats or added carbohydrates.

Supplementation When Required:

For individuals exhibiting particular deficiencies, the administration of supplements such as vitamin D or iron may be necessary to address these gaps.

It is advisable to seek the counsel of a healthcare professional prior to initiating the use of dietary supplements.

A well-balanced diet that prioritizes both macronutrients and micronutrients is essential for promoting cellular health. By comprehending their functions and ensuring their incorporation into your dietary regimen, you can facilitate energy production, cellular repair, and protection, thereby establishing a foundation for sustained health and vitality.

Antioxidants: The Superheroes of Cellular Health

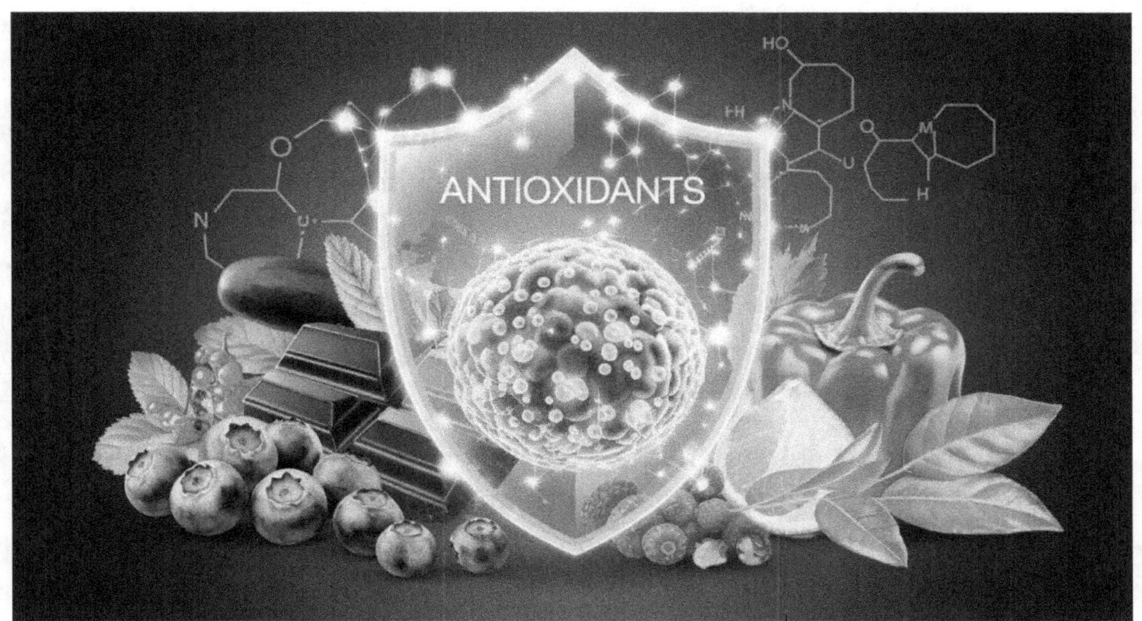

Antioxidants are molecules that play a crucial role in protecting our cells from oxidative stress-induced injury. Antioxidants neutralize free radicals, which are unstable molecules naturally generated during metabolic processes and as a result of exposure to environmental stressors such as pollution, ultraviolet (UV) radiation, and tobacco use. If left unregulated, free radicals have the potential to induce cellular damage, expedite the aging process, and play a role in the development of chronic diseases, including cancer, diabetes, and cardiovascular disorders.

By mitigating oxidative stress, antioxidants serve as the unrecognized champions of cellular health, safeguarding the integrity of cell membranes, DNA, and organelles.

Understanding Free Radicals and Oxidative Stress

What Are Free Radicals?

Free radicals are extremely reactive species characterized by the presence of an unpaired electron. In order to achieve stability, they "extract" electrons from other molecules within our cells, thereby initiating a cascade of cellular injury.

Origins of Free Radicals:

Internal: Standard metabolic processes include the synthesis of adenosine triphosphate (ATP) within the mitochondria.

External factors include pollution, tobacco smoke, alcoholic beverages, ultraviolet radiation, and processed food products.

Oxidative Stress

Oxidative stress arises when the generation of free radicals surpasses the body's capacity to neutralize them through antioxidants. This imbalance has the potential to compromise proteins, lipids, and DNA, thereby disrupting cellular function and possibly resulting in disease.

How Antioxidants Work

Antioxidants stabilize free radicals by donating an electron while maintaining their own stability. This interrupts the cascade of cellular injury and contributes to the preservation of cellular integrity.

Principal Functions of Antioxidants:

- Safeguarding DNA against mutations
- We are mitigating lipid peroxidation, which adversely affects cellular membranes.
- It enhances the immune system's performance by reducing inflammation.

Types of Antioxidants

Antioxidants manifest in various forms, each possessing distinct properties and functions. We can categorize them as endogenous, synthesized by the body, or exogenous, acquired through dietary intake.

1. Endogenous Antioxidants

The human body synthesizes its own antioxidants, which are essential for protection against oxidative stress.

- *Glutathione:* Referred to as the "master antioxidant," it effectively neutralizes free radicals and facilitates the regeneration of other antioxidants, such as vitamins C and E.
- *Superoxide Dismutase (SOD):* Catalyzes the conversion of superoxide radicals into less deleterious molecules.
- *Catalase:* Catalyzes the decomposition of hydrogen peroxide into water and oxygen, thereby mitigating potential cellular damage.

2. Exogenous Antioxidants

Dietary sources provide these nutrients, which are crucial for reestablishing the body's immune defenses.

- *Vitamin C* is a water-soluble antioxidant that safeguards the aqueous environments of cells and enhances collagen synthesis.
  Citrus fruits, strawberries, bell peppers, and broccoli are present.
- *Vitamin E:* A lipophilic antioxidant that protects cellular membranes from oxidative injury.
  Present in: Nuts, seeds, spinach, and sunflower oil.
- *Beta-Carotene and Vitamin A:* Facilitate cellular differentiation and bolster immune health.
  Carrots, sweet potatoes, and apricots are present.
- *Polyphenols:* Phytochemical constituents characterized by robust antioxidant properties.
  Green tea contains catechins, red wine contains resveratrol, and dark chocolate contains flavonoids.
- *Selenium* is a trace mineral that augments the efficacy of endogenous antioxidants, such as glutathione.
  Present: Brazil nuts, eggs, and tuna.

Benefits of Antioxidants for Cellular Health

Protecting DNA: Antioxidants such as vitamin C and selenium mitigate DNA mutations induced by oxidative stress, thereby diminishing the likelihood of cancer and age-related ailments.

Preservation of Cell Membranes: Lipid peroxidation refers to a biochemical process in which free radicals inflict injury upon cell membranes. Antioxidants, such as vitamin E, play a crucial role in preventing this phenomenon by preserving cellular integrity.

Enhancing Mitochondrial Function: The free radicals produced during the process of energy generation within mitochondria have the potential to compromise their functionality. Antioxidants alleviate this issue, thereby facilitating the efficient production of ATP.

Enhancing Immunity: Oxidative stress has the potential to compromise the functionality of immune cells. Antioxidants bolster the body's resilience, thereby augmenting its capacity to combat infections.

Reducing Inflammation: Numerous diseases are associated with chronic inflammation, which oxidative stress exacerbates. Antioxidants mitigate this effect, thereby facilitating cellular repair and enhancing longevity.

Foods Rich in Antioxidants

Fruits and Vegetables

A diet abundant in vibrant fruits and vegetables represents the most effective means of enhancing antioxidant consumption.

- *Berries*, including blueberries, raspberries, and blackberries, are abundant in anthocyanins and vitamin C.
- *Citrus fruits*, such as oranges, lemons, and grapefruits, are excellent sources of vitamin C.
- *Leafy Greens*: Spinach, kale, and Swiss chard are rich sources of lutein and zeaxanthin.

- *Cruciferous vegetables*, such as broccoli and Brussels sprouts, enhance the levels of glutathione.

Nuts and seeds.

Abundant in vitamin E and selenium, they provide robust defense against oxidative damage.

Illustrations include almonds, hazelnuts, flaxseeds, and chia seeds.

Beverages

Certain beverages serve as significant sources of antioxidants.

- *Green Tea:* The catechins present in green tea possess potent antioxidant properties.
- Chlorogenic acid, a potent antioxidant, enhances *coffee.*
- *Red Wine:* Resveratrol, a compound present in red wine, contributes to cellular longevity when consumed in moderation.

Lifestyle Tips to Maximize Antioxidant Benefits

Consume a Diverse Array of Colors: Integrate a wide range of vibrant fruits and vegetables into your diet to guarantee a comprehensive assortment of antioxidants.

Opt for Whole Foods Instead of Supplements: Although supplements may offer assistance, whole foods deliver antioxidants in their natural state, frequently accompanied by synergistic nutrients.

Mitigate Antioxidant Depletion: - Minimize exposure to sources of free radicals, including tobacco use, processed food consumption, and excessive ultraviolet radiation from sun exposure.

Combine Antioxidant-Dense Foods with Nutritious Fats: Fat-soluble antioxidants, such as vitamin E, exhibit enhanced absorption when consumed in conjunction with healthful fats, such as olive oil or avocado.

A Simple Antioxidant-Rich Meal Plan

Breakfast

- *Greek yogurt topped with blueberries, almonds, and a drizzle of honey.*

Lunch

- *Spinach salad with grilled salmon, avocado, cherry tomatoes, and olive oil dressing.*

Snack

- *A handful of walnuts and a green tea latte.*

Dinner

- *Grilled chicken breast with roasted sweet potatoes, steamed broccoli, and a side of quinoa.*

Dessert

- *A square of dark chocolate (70% cocoa or higher).*

Antioxidants constitute a vital defense mechanism that safeguards our cells from the detrimental impacts of free radicals. By integrating a diverse array of antioxidant-rich foods into your diet and reducing oxidative stress, you enhance your body's capacity to sustain cellular health, foster longevity, and avert chronic diseases. These champions of cellular health serve as a reminder that nutrition transcends mere sustenance; it is a potent instrument for both healing and safeguarding the body.

Key Foods for Cellular Repair and Energy Boosting

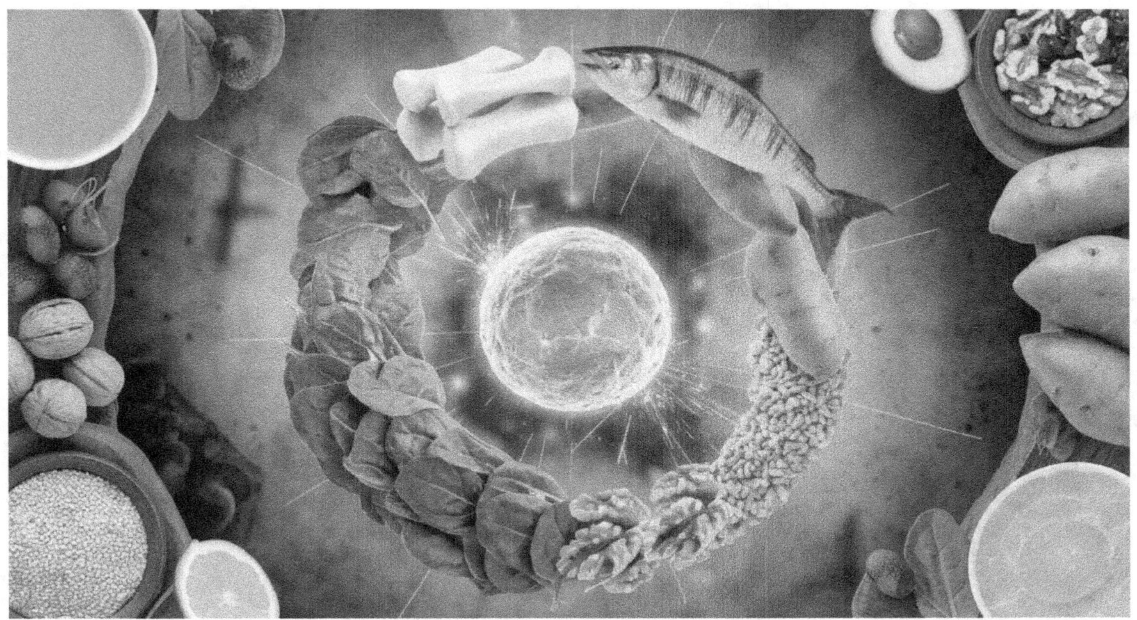

The foods we consume play a crucial role in our body's capacity to repair damaged cells, regenerate new ones, and generate energy for daily activities. A meticulously structured diet, abundant in particular nutrients, can facilitate cellular repair and optimize energy production, thereby promoting overall health and vitality. Let us examine the fundamental nutrients and their influence on these vital cellular processes.

Why Cellular Repair and Energy Boosting Matter

Cellular Repair: Cells experience daily degradation as a result of physical exertion, exposure to harmful substances, oxidative stress, and the intrinsic process of aging. Nutritional substances that facilitate repair contribute to the preservation of tissue integrity, the prevention of maladies, and the deceleration of the aging process.

Energy Production: Cellular energy, which takes the form of adenosine triphosphate (ATP), powers all physiological processes in the body, including cognition and movement. Nutrient-dense diets facilitate optimal mitochondrial function, the site of energy production.

Categories of Foods for Cellular Restoration and Energy Enhancement

Foods High in Protein:

Proteins play a crucial role in cellular restoration and regeneration, as they supply amino acids, which serve as the fundamental components of cellular structures, enzymes, and hormones.

Key Foods:

- *Eggs* serve as a comprehensive source of protein, encompassing all nine essential amino acids.
- *Lean meats*, such as chicken, turkey, and beef, provide a superior source of protein essential for the repair of muscle and tissue.
- *Fish* such as salmon, tuna, and mackerel are abundant sources of protein and omega-3 fatty acids, which are known to mitigate inflammation and facilitate cellular repair.
- *Plant-Based Proteins*: Lentils, lentils, tofu, and quinoa serve as exceptional sources of protein for individuals adhering to vegetarian and vegan diets.

Nutritional Highlights:

- *Amino acids*, such as leucine found in eggs and meat, promote the repair of muscle and tissue.
- *Collagen,* as found in bone broth, facilitates the regeneration of cells in both the epidermis and joints.

Healthy Fats: The Protectors

The Guardians Lipids, particularly omega-3 fatty acids, play a crucial role in cellular repair and the generation of energy. They contribute to the preservation of cell membrane integrity and mitigate inflammation.

Key Foods

- *Fatty fish*, such as salmon, sardines, and trout, are rich sources of omega-3 fatty acids, specifically docosahexaenoic acid (DHA) and eicosapentaenoic acid (EPA).
- *Avocados* are rich in monounsaturated lipids and antioxidants, which contribute to cellular protection.
- *Nuts and seeds*, including almonds, walnuts, flaxseeds, and chia seeds, provide beneficial lipids and vitamin E, which contribute to the repair of cellular membranes.
- *Olive oil*, which is abundant in oleic acid, contributes to anti-inflammatory mechanisms.

Nutritional Highlights:

- *Omega-3 fatty acids* facilitate the repair of neuronal cells and contribute to cardiovascular well-being.
- *Vitamin E* present in almonds serves to protect cells from oxidative stress.

Foods Rich in Antioxidants:

The Guardians Antioxidants protect cells from free radical-induced oxidative damage and aid in the repair of damaged DNA and tissues.

Key Foods

- *Berries*, including blueberries, raspberries, and blackberries, are abundant in anthocyanins, which are potent antioxidants.
- *Leafy greens,* such as spinach and kale, are rich in lutein, zeaxanthin, and beta-carotene, which contribute to cellular health.
- *Citrus fruits*, such as oranges, lemons, and grapefruits, are rich sources of vitamin C, which is essential for the synthesis of collagen.
- *Tomatoes* are rich in lycopene, a compound that serves to safeguard cells against ultraviolet damage.

- *Dark Chocolate:* The flavonoids present in dark chocolate enhance mitochondrial function and promote increased blood flow to cells.

Nutritional Highlights:

- *Vitamin C* facilitates tissue repair and bolsters immune function.
- Studies have shown that the *polyphenols* in berries and green tea can reduce cellular inflammation.

Whole Grains and Complex Carbohydrates: The Energizers

Carbohydrates serve as the principal source of energy for the body, facilitating cellular respiration within the mitochondria to generate adenosine triphosphate (ATP). Complex carbohydrates facilitate a gradual release of glucose, thereby providing sustained energy.

Key Foods

- *Oats:* Offer soluble fiber and a gradual release of energy.
- *Quinoa* is considered a complete protein because it contains all essential amino acids and complex carbohydrates.
- *Sweet potatoes* are rich in beta-carotene and provide energy-enhancing carbohydrates.
- *Brown rice* is a source of manganese, a mineral that plays a crucial role in energy metabolism.

Nutritional Highlights:

- Complex carbohydrates produce *glucose,* which is the primary substrate for the synthesis of cellular energy.
- *B vitamins* present in whole grains facilitate the pathways involved in energy metabolism.

Iron-Rich Foods: The Oxygen Carriers

Iron is essential for the synthesis of hemoglobin, which facilitates the transport of oxygen to cells for the purpose of energy production. In the absence of adequate oxygen, cells are unable to synthesize adenosine triphosphate (ATP) effectively.

Key Foods:

- The human body readily absorbs heme iron, which is abundant in *red meat.*
- *Spinach* provides non-heme iron, which is particularly beneficial when consumed in conjunction with vitamin C.
- *Leguminous plants:* Lentils, chickpeas, and legumes serve as plant-derived sources of iron.
- *Fortified Cereals* are a convenient method to enhance iron consumption.

Highlights of Nutritional Value:

- *Iron* plays a crucial role in supporting mitochondrial function and facilitating energy metabolism.
- Foods abundant in *vitamin C*, such as oranges, facilitate the assimilation of iron.

Foods Rich in B Vitamins

The Catalysts B vitamins serve as crucial cofactors in the processes of energy production and cellular repair.

Key Foods

- *Eggs and dairy* products are abundant sources of vitamin B2 (riboflavin) and vitamin B12, both of which play a crucial role in energy metabolism.
- *Whole grains* serve as a source of vitamin B1 (thiamine) and vitamin B3 (niacin), both of which are essential for the production of adenosine triphosphate (ATP).
- *Leafy greens*, such as spinach and kale, serve as excellent sources of folate (vitamin B9).
- *Poultry*, specifically chicken and turkey, provides vitamin B6, which is essential for the synthesis of neurotransmitters.

Highlights of Nutritional Value:

- *B vitamins* function as essential cofactors in the Krebs cycle, facilitating the production of adenosine triphosphate (ATP).
- *Folate (B9)* is essential for the synthesis and repair of DNA.

Foods Rich in Zinc and Selenium: The Repair Catalysts

Zinc and selenium are essential elements that significantly contribute to tissue repair and the functioning of the immune system.

Key Foods

- *Oysters and shellfish* are rich in zinc, an essential mineral that plays a crucial role in the process of wound repair.
- *Brazil nuts* serve as a substantial source of selenium, an antioxidant that facilitates cellular repair.
- *Pumpkin seeds* are a source of both zinc and magnesium, contributing to cellular health.
- *Mushrooms* are a source of selenium and various other micronutrients.

Highlights of Nutritional Value:

- *Zinc* facilitates the synthesis of enzymes essential for cellular repair.
- *Selenium* serves to mitigate oxidative damage and facilitates the repair of DNA.

Hydrating Foods:

The Facilitators of Transport Adequate hydration is crucial for cellular functions, encompassing the transportation of nutrients and the elimination of waste products.

Key Foods

- *Cucumber:* Its elevated water content contributes significantly to the maintenance of hydration.

- *Watermelon* provides hydration and is a rich source of antioxidants, including lycopene.
- *Coconut water:* Its natural electrolytes enhance cellular hydration.

Nutritional Highlights:

- *Appropriate hydration* facilitates energy metabolism.
- *Electrolytes* play a crucial role in maintaining the balance of cellular fluids.

Integrating Key Foods into Your Diet

Breakfast: *Greek yogurt with blueberries, chia seeds, and a drizzle of honey.*

Lunch: *Grilled salmon with quinoa, sautéed spinach, and avocado.*

Snack: *A handful of almonds and a green tea.*

Dinner: *Lean chicken breast with roasted sweet potatoes and steamed broccoli.*

Dessert: *A square of dark chocolate paired with fresh strawberries.*

Essential foods that promote cellular repair and enhance energy levels supply vital nutrients that support the body's inherent regeneration mechanisms and energy synthesis. By integrating a varied assortment of these foods into your diet, you not only promote the integrity and longevity of your cells but also augment your overall vitality and fortitude against disease. This dietary approach emphasizes the significant relationship between nutrition and cellular well-being, enabling individuals to flourish from within.

CHAPTER 5

CELLULAR DETOXIFICATION – HOW TO CLEANSE AND REVITALIZE YOUR CELLS

There is more to cellular cleansing than just getting rid of toxins. Giving your cells a fresh start allows them to function optimally, produce energy efficiently, and repair any stress-inducing factors such as pollution, processed foods, and waste products from your body. Your body's natural healing processes will work better, your vitality will rise, and your general health will get better. For a better, more energetic life, here's how to clean and spark up your cells.

Staying Hydrated Is The First Step In Detoxification.

Water is an important part of the cleansing process. It gets rid of waste, brings nutrients to cells, and keeps cells working at their best. Being hydrated is important for all of your body's functions, like digestion, circulation, and cleansing.

Staying hydrated is important for cellular health because water helps move toxins to the kidneys so they can be flushed out of the body.

- It keeps the blood flowing properly, which is needed to get nutrients to cells.
- It helps maintain the balance of fluids inside cells, which is crucial for their ability to function.

To stay hydrated, drink at least 2 liters (8 cups) of water every day.

- Putting lemon in your water first thing in the morning will help your body clean.
- Teas with herbs, like mint or ginger, are also excellent ways to stay hydrated.

- Think about eating foods that are high in water, like oranges, cucumbers, and tomatoes.

Improve Gut Health for Efficient Detoxification

People often call the gut the "second brain" because it is essential for defense, absorbing nutrients, and getting rid of waste. Having a healthy gut helps your body get rid of trash and toxins.

Why Gut Health is Important for Detox:

- A healthy gut microbiome helps break down toxins and receive nutrients for healing and energy production.
- The lining of the gut prevents harmful chemicals from entering the bloodstream.
- Leaky gut syndrome can happen when your gut isn't healthy. Toxins can get into your bloodstream and make you feel sick.

To Improve Gut Health

- Eat foods that are high in probiotics. For example, yogurt, kefir, sauerkraut, kimchi, and miso can help restore healthy bugs.
- Eat fiber. Fiber keeps you from getting constipated and helps move toxins through your digestive system. Eat things like apples, beans, chia seeds, and oats.
- Hydrate: Water is also important for gut health because it helps keep bowel movements normal.

Eat Detoxifying Foods

Certain foods naturally cleanse the body, aid in the removal of waste, and aid in the repair of damaged cells. These foods give you important nutrients and vitamins that keep cells from getting hurt by free radicals.

Cruciferous Vegetables:

- Crispy vegetables include broccoli, cauliflower, kale, Brussels sprouts, and more.

- The sulfur compounds in these vegetables aid the liver in breaking down and eliminating toxins.

Leafy Greens:

- Spinach, mustard greens, and arugula are some examples.
- Leafy veggies help get rid of toxins from the body because they contain chlorophyll. They also help the liver's cleaning processes.

Beets:

- Beets are full of vitamins and help the liver get rid of waste by making more bile flow.

Lemon:

- Lemons are full of vitamin C, which helps the liver's cleansing enzymes work better. In the morning, drinking lemon water helps your body digest food and get rid of waste.

Garlic:

- Garlic contains sulfur molecules that enhance the function of liver enzymes, thereby aiding in liver cleansing and improving detoxification.

Berries:

- Strawberries, blueberries, and raspberries are all full of antioxidants that protect cells from damage caused by oxidative stress.

Help The Liver Work

The liver is the body's main organ for cleansing, and making it work better is important for cleaning out cells. It gets rid of dangerous substances in the blood, breaks down toxins, and processes waste.

Foods That Help The Liver Detox:

- Curcumin, which is found in turmeric, helps lower inflammation and supports the activity of liver enzymes.
- Milk thistle helps the liver heal and clean itself out better.
- Green tea has a lot of catechins, which are good for your liver and help your body burn fat.
- Avocados: They help the liver make glutathione, which is a strong antioxidant that helps the body get rid of toxins.

Habits for a Healthy Liver:

- Don't drink too much booze, as it can put stress on the liver.
- Eat less prepared foods and trans fats, which can make your liver swell up.
- Doing regular physical activity helps keep liver enzymes in check and stops fat from building up in the liver.

Try Intermittent Fasting

Intermittent fasting (IF) means going back and forth between eating and not eating. This practice not only lowers the amount of toxins you take in, but it also speeds up cell repair processes like autophagy.

Autophagy and Cellular Detox:

- Autophagy is the process by which the body gets rid of broken or useless cells and replaces them with new ones. This renews cells and gets rid of toxins.
- When you fast, your body goes into a state where it saves energy and repairs broken cells while getting rid of toxins.

Different kinds of intermittent fasting:

- 16/8 Method: Don't eat for 16 hours and then eat within an 8-hour window.
- If you do alternate day fasting, you don't eat or drink anything every other day.

- Eat-Stop-Eat: Once or twice a week, don't eat for 24 hours.
- Time-Restricted Eating: Make sure your eating habits match your body's natural cycles, which can help your metabolism and clean.

Exercise regularly to help the Body Detox

Being active makes you sweat, which is an important way for the body to get rid of toxins. It also makes the blood flow faster, which helps toxins get to the liver and kidneys to be processed and flushed out of the body.

How Exercise Helps:

- It raises blood flow, which brings oxygen and nutrients to tissues and helps get rid of waste.
- Encourages Sweating: Toxins like heavy metals and bisphenol A (BPA) are flushed out of the body through sweat
- Improves Lymphatic Flow: Regular movement wakes up the lymphatic system, which helps the immune system work and gets rid of trash

Tips for Working Out:

- Aim for at least 30 minutes of mild exercise most days of the week.
- For the best circulation and detox benefits, do both aerobic activities (like running and swimming) and strength training (like yoga and lifting weights).

Get Enough Good Sleep

Getting enough sleep is an important part of detoxifying cells. The body fixes and renews cells, gets rid of waste from the brain, and cleans out tissues while you sleep. On the other hand, not getting enough sleep raises stress chemicals like cortisol, which can damage cells.

Why Getting Enough Sleep Is Good For Detox:

- Brain Detoxification: While you sleep, the brain's glymphatic system gets rid of toxins like beta-amyloid plaques that are linked to neurological illnesses.
- Cellular fix: While you sleep, your body makes more growth hormone, which helps fix tissues and make cells younger.

Tips for Better Sleep:

- Aim for 7–9 hours of good sleep every night.
- Make a relaxing routine for the evening to lower your stress and get a better night's sleep (for example, stay away from screens and practice relaxation methods).
- Go to bed and wake up at the same time every day to keep a regular sleep routine.

Understanding Cellular Toxins and Their Impact

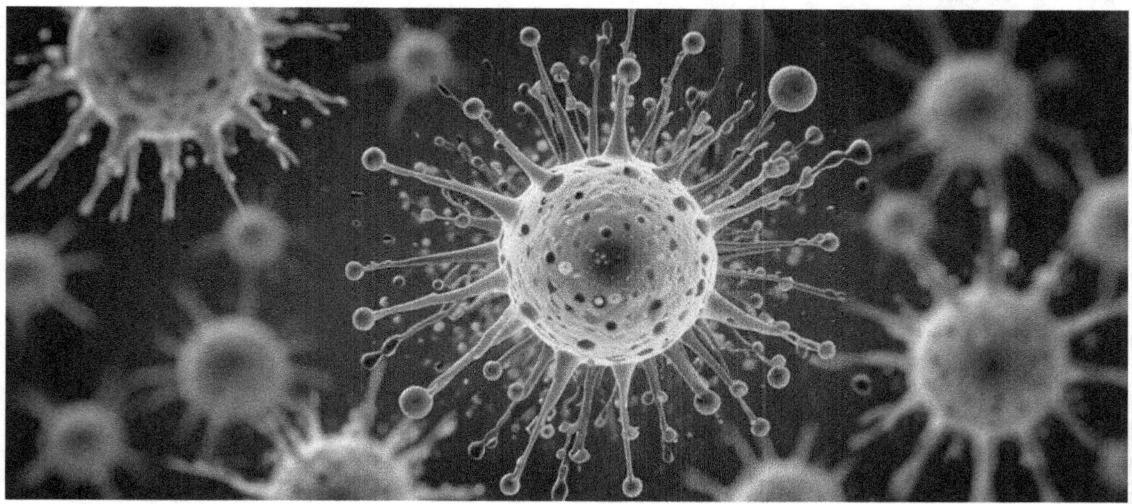

Toxins are chemicals and other substances that can stop your cells from working normally. They are everywhere in today's world. From your environment, food, or metabolic processes, these toxins can build up and damage your cells. To stay healthy and avoid getting sick, you need to know how toxins affect your cells and what you can do to lessen their effects.

This section describes cellular toxins, how they disrupt cell function, and how to avoid them.

What Are Cellular Toxins?

There are harmful chemicals called cellular toxins that stop your cells from working normally. These toxins can come from inside the body (endogenous) or outside the body (exogenous). They can hurt parts of cells, mess up biochemical processes, and make it harder for the body to heal itself. More and more toxins build up inside cells over time, which leads to chronic diseases, early aging, and less energy.

Types of Cellular Toxins

Toxins made by the body (Endogenous Toxins)

Ordinary biological processes inside the body produce toxins like these. As an example:

- Reactive Oxygen Species (ROS) are byproducts of cellular respiration that can cause reactive stress if there are too many of them.
- When you exercise vigorously and don't get enough air, you produce lactic acid.
- Metabolic waste products, such as urea and ammonia, require immediate disposal to prevent harm.

Exogenous Toxins:

These toxins come from outside sources, like food, surroundings, and ways of life. Some examples are

- The land, water, and air all contain certain chemicals and pollutants.

- Lead, mercury, and arsenic are examples of extremely heavy metals.
- Normal food cultivation involves the use of pesticides and herbicides.
- Processed foods have extra ingredients, chemicals that keep them fresh, and fake ones.
- Medications and drugs: Certain prescription drugs and recreational drugs can overwork the body's cleansing systems.

How Toxins Affect Cellular Functions

Toxins can disrupt the functioning of cells in various ways, leading to damage and issues throughout the body. In order, here are the main ways that toxins hurt your cells:

Oxidative Stress

What is oxidative stress?

When there is an imbalance in the body between free radicals (molecules that are not stable) and antioxidants, oxidative stress happens. Free radicals can damage DNA, proteins, and lipids inside cells because they are very reactive.

How Toxins Contribute

Many toxins, like heavy metals and chemicals, make more free radicals. This causes ongoing oxidative stress over time, which makes diseases like cancer, Alzheimer's, and heart disease more likely.

Problems With The Mitochondria

The Mitochondria's Job:

The mitochondria are the cells' power plants; they make ATP, which is the body's energy exchange. For energy output and cell repair, mitochondria must be in excellent health.

How toxins interfere:

Toxins such as alcohol, pesticides, and some medicines damage mitochondria, causing them to function less effectively, leading to fatigue, mental fog, and muscle weakness.

Interruption of Signaling in Cells

Cellular communication is necessary to keep homeostasis and make sure that reactions to stress or injury work together.

Effects of toxins: Some toxins, such as endocrine disruptors (like BPA and phthalates), disrupt the communication between hormones. This can cause changes that affect metabolism, growth, and reproduction.

Inflammation:

Toxins often set off the immune system, which causes long-lasting inflammation. Short-term inflammation protects tissues, but long-term inflammation hurts them and speeds up cell aging and illness.

Detoxification Problems:

Toxins build up faster than the body can get rid of them, and the detoxification routes get too busy to work properly. Toxins build up in tissues and organs because of this, which makes cell damage even worse.

Different kinds of Cellular Toxins

Below is a list of some of the most common toxins that harm cell health.

Heavy Metals

- Lead, mercury, arsenic, and cadmium are some examples.
- Sources include polluted water, certain seafood such as tuna and swordfish, and pollution from factories.
- The DNA, nervous system, and mitochondria suffer damage.

Pesticides and Herbicides

- Glyphosate and organophosphates are two examples.
- Sources: Fruits, veggies, and grains grown in factory farms.
- Hormonal imbalances, toxic stress, and a weak immune system are some of the effects.

Pollutants in the Environment

- Particulates in the air, industrial chemicals, and plastics are some examples.
- Sources: Plastics, home goods, and air pollution.
- The effects include long-term inflammation and breathing problems.

Additives and Preservatives for Food

- Artificial sugar, MSG, and trans fats are some examples.
- The sources are processed or packed foods.
- The effects include alterations in the gut flora, inflammation, and the utilization of energy.

Tobacco and Alcohol

- Sources: cigarettes, alcoholic drinks, and smoking gear.
- The effects include harm to the liver, oxidative stress, and DNA damage.

The Body's Detoxification System

Your body has built-in systems for getting rid of and removing toxins, but these systems can get overworked when the body is exposed to too many.

The Liver

The liver is the primary organ responsible for eliminating toxins. The liver transforms toxins that dissolve in fat into forms that dissolve in water, which the body can flush out through urine or bile.

One important nutrient for liver cleansing is glutathione, which is a strong antioxidant.

Vitamins B6, B12, and folate

Consume foods rich in sulfur, such as onions and garlic.

The Kidneys

The kidneys remove waste and toxins from the blood and flush them out of the body through pee.

Staying hydrated can help your kidneys get rid of waste.

Consuming high-potassium foods such as bananas and avocados is beneficial.

The Lymphatic System:

The lymphatic system helps move waste and toxins out of the body's cells.

Exercise, dry brushing, and deep breathing can help the lymphatic system work better, which can improve detoxification.

Cellular Autophagy:

Autophagy is how cells get rid of broken parts and toxins.

Fasting, exercise, and a healthy diet can all help autophagy happen, which helps cells clean up and heal.

What Cellular Toxins Do to Your Health

When poisons build up in your cells, they can cause many health problems, such as

Chronic Diseases:

Toxins cause inflammation, oxidative stress, and DNA damage, all of which play a role in chronic diseases like diabetes, heart disease, and cancer.

Neurodegenerative Disorders

Brain diseases that get worse over time: Researchers have linked Alzheimer's, Parkinson's, and other brain diseases to heavy metals and toxins in the environment.

Immune Dysfunction

Toxins weaken the immune system, which makes the body more likely to get illnesses and autoimmune diseases.

Aging too quickly:

Toxins cause oxidative stress, which speeds up the aging process of cells. This can cause wrinkles, less energy, and diseases that come with getting older.

Supporting Cellular Detoxification

Consider the following ways to keep your cells safe from chemicals and help with detoxification:

Limit your Exposure To Toxins.

- To cut down on pesticides, choose organic foods.
- Stay away from prepared foods and added chemicals.
- Clean and care for yourself with natural, non-toxic items.

Eat Foods That Help Your Body Detox.

- Cruciferous veggies, like broccoli and kale, can help your liver get rid of toxins.

- To fight oxidative stress, eat foods that are high in antioxidants, such as berries, green tea, and ginger.

Stay Hydrated:

- Drink a lot of water to help your kidneys work well and get rid of waste through pee.

Take Care Of Your Gut Health.

- A favorable gut microbiome is an important part of detoxification. To keep your gut healthy, eat foods that are high in fiber and bacteria, like yogurt and kefir.

Do a Lot Of Physical Exercise.

- Being active improves circulation, lymphatic drainage, and mitochondrial function, all of which help the body get rid of toxins.

Choose Vitamins Wisely:

- To help the body's detoxification processes, think about taking vitamins like milk thistle, NAC (N-acetylcysteine), and glutathione.

Modern life is full of cellular toxins, but you can lessen their effects by making wise decisions and exercising caution. You can protect the health of your cells, lower your risk of chronic disease, and improve your general vitality by learning how toxins affect your cells and taking steps to help detoxification. We will talk about how diet, lifestyle, and targeted interventions can improve cellular health and resilience in the next parts.

Detox-Friendly Foods and Supplements

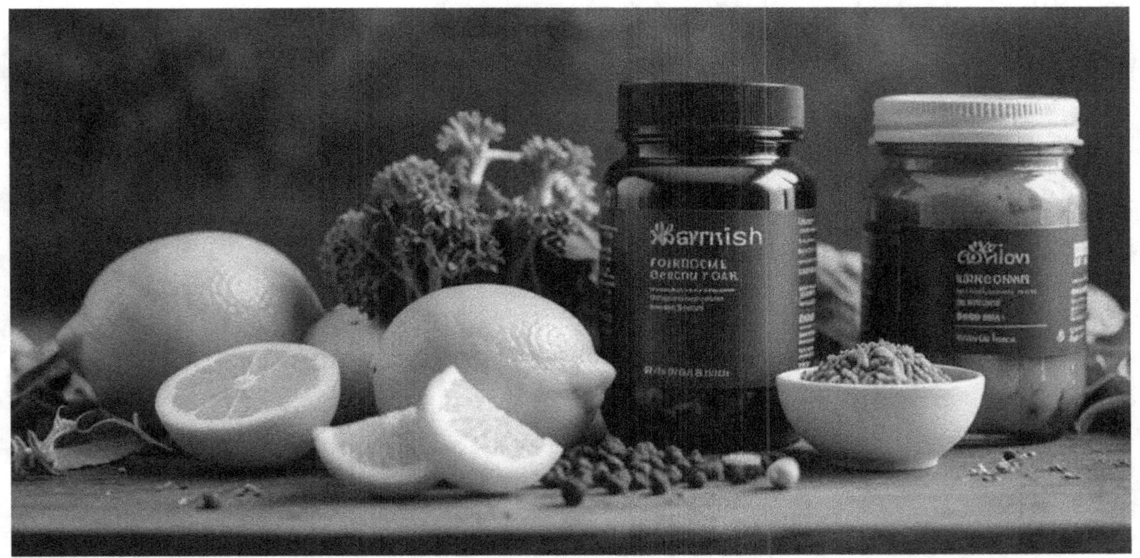

The body naturally detoxifies itself, but you can support and speed up the process by eating certain foods and taking vitamins that help get rid of toxins, fix damage, and make cells work better. These vitamins and foods not only help clean the body, but they also feed and protect cells so they work at their best.

Foods that are Beneficial For Detoxing

There are foods that are known to help the liver, kidneys, gut, and other detox processes. By adding these things to your diet, you can help your body clean itself naturally.

Leafy Greens with Crucifers

- Broccoli, cauliflower, Brussels sprouts, kale, and cabbage are some examples.
- How They Work: They contain glucosinolates, which are chemicals that assist liver enzymes in eliminating harmful substances.
- Key Benefit: Promote healthy liver function and aid in the removal of toxins through bile.

Leafy Greens:

- Swiss chard, spinach, arugula, and dandelion greens are all examples.
- How They Work: Their high chlorophyll content prevents the body's digestive system from absorbing toxins.
- Key Benefit: Improve digestion and keep the liver healthy.

Citrus Fruits

- Include limes, lemons, oranges, and grapefruits. How They Work:
- They are high in vitamin C, which raises glutathione levels.
- Glutathione is a main antioxidant that helps the body get rid of toxins. They improve immune function and enzyme activity in the liver.

Beets

- They are high in betalains and antioxidants, which help liver enzymes work and bile production.
- They also help break down poisons and get rid of them from the body.

Onions and Garlic

- How They Work: Their sulfur compounds stimulate the liver enzymes to eliminate toxins.
- Key Benefits: They enhance the immune system and aid in liver cleansing.

Berries:

- Blackberries, blueberries, and strawberries are some examples.
- How They Work: They're full of antioxidants that fight free radicals and lower inflammation.
- The primary benefit is to shield cells from the oxidative damage that toxins cause.

Spices and Herbs

- Turmeric, ginger, cilantro, and parsley are some examples.
- How They Work: o The curcumin found in turmeric improves liver function and reduces inflammation.
- Cilantro helps the body get rid of heavy metals.
- Ginger helps your body digest food and improves blood flow.
- Key benefit: Offer a variety of cleansing methods.

Foods That Keep You Hydrated

- Cucumbers, tomatoes, and celery are all examples.
- How They Work: They give you water and minerals to flush out toxins and keep your cells hydrated.
- Key Benefit: Help the kidneys work better and keep your skin healthy.

Supplements that Help Detox

Food should be your main source of nutrients, but pills can help when your body needs extra help detoxing or when the nutrients in your food aren't enough.

Milk Thistle:

- Its active ingredient, silymarin, aids in the regeneration of liver cells and enhances the liver's detoxification capabilities.
- How to Use It: Follow the directions and take between 200 and 400 mg per day.

Probiotics:

- Helps keep the bacteria in your gut healthy, which helps digestion and keeps harmful substances from getting into your bloodstream.
- You should consume them as pills or in fermented foods like kimchi and yogurt.

Glutathione:

- How It Works: Glutathione is the body's main antioxidant. It gets rid of toxins straight and helps the liver work.
- You can take it as a vitamin or as the precursor N-acetylcysteine (NAC).

Chlorella and Spirulina

- How They Work: Supplements made from algae bind to heavy metals and toxins and help the body get rid of them through digestion.
- Powders or capsules should be a part of your daily practice.

Activated Charcoal:

- How it works: it binds to toxins in the gut and stops them from being absorbed.
- How to use it: for a short-term clean under the supervision of a doctor.

Healthy Fats (omega-3)

- How They Work: They lower inflammation and improve the health of cell membranes, which helps the body's detoxification processes.
- Fish oil pills or fatty fish such as salmon are the best ways to achieve this.

The Role of Fasting and Intermittent Fasting

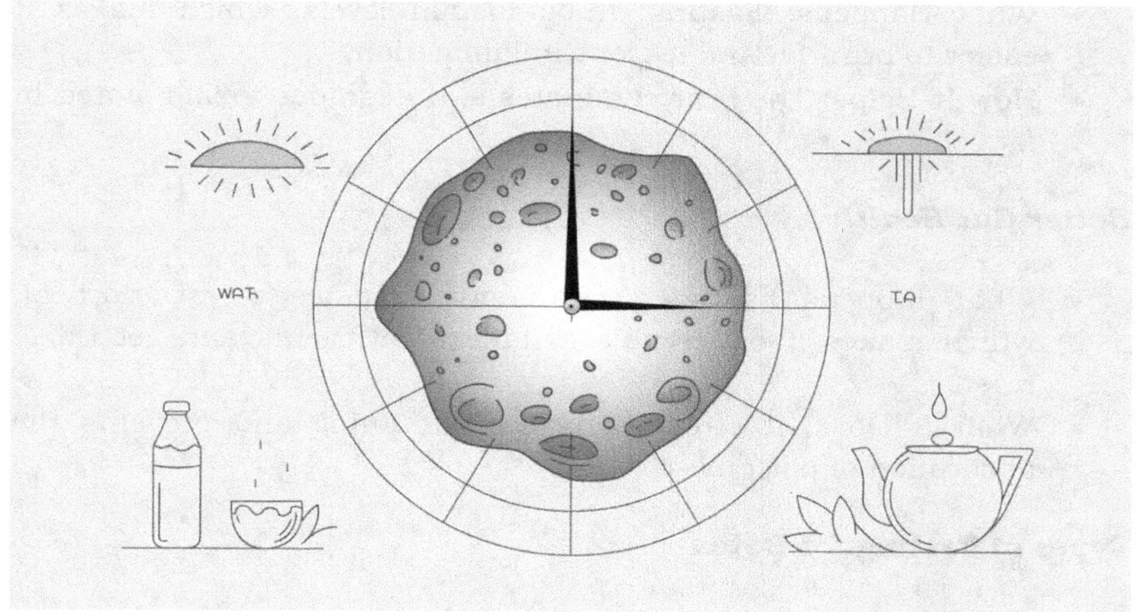

Fasting is one of the best ways to get rid of toxins. When the body isn't busy processing food, it can use its energy to fix cells, get rid of waste, and make the whole system work better.

How Fasting Can Help With Detoxification

When you fast, your body's metabolism changes in a number of ways that have a direct effect on cleansing.

Autophagy

What is autophagy? It's a process in cells that gets rid of old, broken, or useless parts and reuses them.

What It Does:

- Gets rid of dangerous toxins in cells.
- It stimulates the repair and renewal of cells
- It effectively prevents inflammation and reactive stress.

Less Insulin In The Blood

- What Happens: Fasting drops insulin levels, which makes it easier to burn fat and lessens inflammation.
- How It Helps: The liver eliminates and degrades toxins stored in fat cells.

Better Gut Health

- What Happens: Fasting gives the gut a chance to rest and heal, which makes it better able to take in nutrients and get rid of trash.
- What It Does: It strengthens the gut lining and prevents the absorption of poisons.

Types of Fasting for Detox

There are different ways to fast, and each has its own perks. Here are some common methods of fasting:

Intermittent Fasting (IF)

- The 16/8 method: don't eat for 16 hours and then eat within an 8-hour window.
- It lowers oxidative stress, speeds up autophagy, and improves metabolic health.

Alternate-Day Fasting

- What It Is: Going without food every other day and eating very few calories on days you don't eat.
- Benefits: Burns more fat and speeds up the cleansing process.

24-Hour Fasts

- What It Is: going without food for a whole day, usually once or twice a week.
- Benefits: It speeds up autophagy and aids in cell healing.

Prolonged Fasting

- It involves not eating or drinking for 48 to 72 hours.
- Benefits: It increases the amount of autophagy and stimulates the growth of immune cells.

Useful Tips for Fastin

Sometimes fasting is hard, especially when you are new to it. To make it easier and work better, do the following:

- Start Slowly: Begin with a 12-hour fast and gradually increase the duration of your fast.
- Stay hydrated: To avoid getting dehydrated, drink a lot of water, herbal teas, or salts.
- Eat meals that are high in nutrients. To fuel your body, break your fast with meals that are high in fiber, protein, and healthy fats.
- Pay attention to your body. If you feel sick, dizzy, or way too tired, stop fasting and see a doctor.
- Get Professional Help: If you want to fast for a long time, talk to a doctor or nurse to make sure you do it safely.

Fasting, detox-friendly foods, and supplements are all powerful ways to support your body's natural detoxification processes and improve the health of your cells. You can clean out your cells, wake up your body, and improve your general health by eating nutrient-dense foods, staying hydrated, and trying out fasting. These tactics, along with living a balanced life, are important parts of a complete plan for long-term health.

CHAPTER 6

THE CELLULAR HEALTH DIET – A BLUEPRINT FOR VITALITY

One of the best ways to fuel cellular health, support vitality, and improve general well-being is with a well-planned diet. Understanding how the food you eat affects the way cells work and incorporating key ideas into your daily life can help you live a healthy life in the long run.

Building a Diet That Fuels Cellular Health

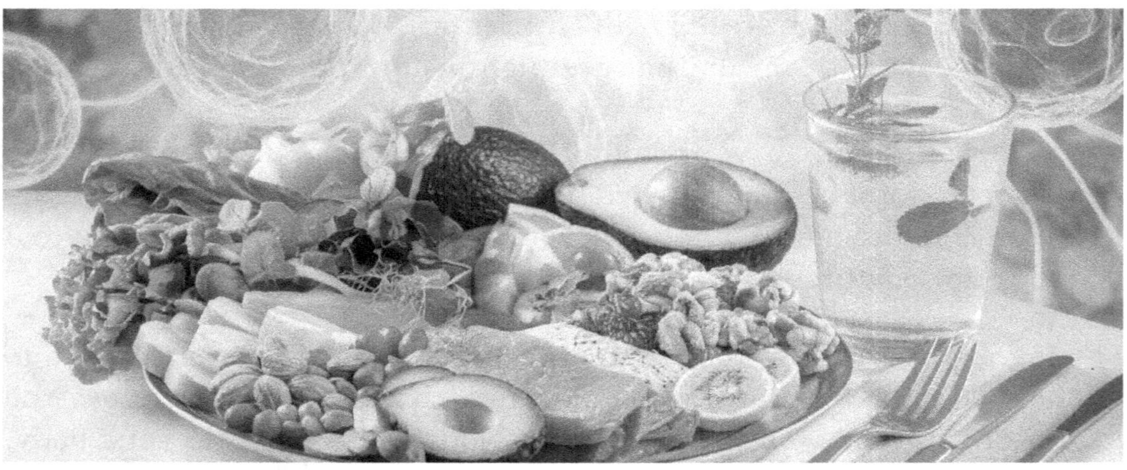

The food you eat has a direct effect on the health and performance of your cells. It changes how they make energy, fix themselves, and work in general. We should minimize toxins and support the processes that optimize cell performance. This is what a diet that focuses on cellular health does. Here is a more in-depth look at how to put together such a plan.

Prioritize Nutrient Density

Foods that are high in nutrients have a lot of vitamins, minerals, and enzymes but not many calories. These chemicals are necessary for many cellular processes:

Vitamins like B-complex (B1, B2, B3, B6, and B12) are essential for breaking down food into energy. Minerals like magnesium and potassium help enzymes work in cells. Antioxidants like vitamin C, vitamin E, and selenium stop free radicals from damaging cells.

Here are some foods that are high in nutrients: Leafy greens like spinach and kale • Fruits with lots of color, like berries and citrus, fish high in fat, such as salmon and sardines, as well as nuts and seeds, such as walnuts, almonds, and chia seeds, are recommended.

Balance Macronutrients to Meet Cellular Needs

Carbs, proteins, and fats are the three main macronutrients. Each of them has a unique role to play in maintaining cell health:

Carbohydrates: Give cells glucose, which is their main source of energy. Choose complex carbs like quinoa, oats, and sweet potatoes. They give you energy slowly and won't cause your blood sugar to rise. Avoid refined sugars and simple carbohydrates. Too much glucose can damage cells and cause inflammation.

Proteins: Your body needs amino acids from proteins to repair cells, produce enzymes, and create new cells. Consume lean foods such as beans, fish, and chicken. For more fiber and less saturated fat, try plant-based meats like tofu, lentils, and tempeh.

Fats: The fats in our food help keep cell walls strong and give us energy over time. Pay attention to good fats such as monounsaturated fats found in avocados and olive oil, and omega-3s found in fish, flaxseeds, and walnuts. Trans fats and hydrogenated oils hurt cell function and make inflammation worse, so eat less of them.

Eat Foods That Lower Inflammation.

Over time, chronic inflammation hurts the structures of cells, making them less able to do their jobs. Anti-inflammatory foods stop dangerous inflammatory pathways from working, which helps fight this.

Foods that reduce inflammation: Foods that are high in omega-3 fatty acids, like fish, turmeric (which has curcumin, a strong anti-inflammatory substance), berries are rich in flavonoids and anthocyanins, and green tea which is high in catechins.

Staying Hydrated Is Important For Cell Health.

Water is an important part of cell activity because it helps move nutrients around, get rid of waste, and keep the structure of cells. Dehydration can make cells less effective, which can affect how they make energy and fix themselves.

Hydration Tips: Aim to drink at least 2 to 3 liters of water every day, but make sure to change this based on how active you are. Eat foods that keep you hydrated, like oranges, cucumbers, and watermelons. Don't drink too much booze or caffeine, which can dry out cells.

Take Care Of Your Gut Health For Better Nutrient Absorption.

How well nutrients are taken and toxins are flushed out of the body depends on how healthy the gut is. A good gut microbiome makes nutrients more available and lowers inflammation.

Gut-healthy foods include probiotics: which are good bacteria that can be found in yogurt, kefir, kimchi, and cabbage. Good bacteria are fed by foods like garlic, onions, bananas, and asparagus.

Fiber-Rich Foods: Vegetables, whole grains, and beans help your body digest food properly and get rid of toxins.

Cut down on Your Intake of Processed Foods causing Toxins.

A lot of processed foods in today's meals are full of chemicals, preservatives, and artificial ingredients that can hurt the health of cells. These foods contain toxins that raise oxidative stress and put a lot of stress on detoxifying pathways.

Avoid or limit these foods: Processed meats (like hot dogs and bacon), snacks and drinks that are high in sugar, sugar substitutes and flavorings, and refined oils (like corn and soybean oil)

Cleaner Food Options: To lower your exposure to pesticides, choose organic food when you can. Choose foods that haven't been changed much, like fresh fruits, veggies, and whole grains. Make your own meals to keep track of what's in them and avoid secret toxins.

Focus on Foods That Are High In Antioxidants.

Antioxidants are very important for keeping cells safe from the damage that free radicals do. A food high in antioxidants makes cells stronger and longer-lasting.

Some of the best foods for antioxidants are: Dark chocolate (with at least 70% cacao); Nuts, especially pecans and walnuts; Artichokes, spinach, and beets.

Eat Foods That Help Cells Heal And Grow.

Some foods, especially those high in zinc, vitamin C, and amino acids, help cells heal themselves better than others.

For example: Bone broth because it has glycine and collagen, which help tissues heal; Citrus fruits are full of vitamin C, which helps your body make more collagen; and Shellfish which are high in zinc needed to repair DNA.

Align Meals with Circadian Rhythms

Eating at times in sync with your body's natural circadian rhythms makes cells work better. Eating during the day helps your body use nutrients better and lowers metabolic stress.

Advice on When to Eat: Eat a healthy breakfast in the morning to get your energy back; Don't eat late at night, because it can stop your cells from healing while you sleep; To give cells time to heal and grow back, think about doing periodic fasting or time-restricted eating.

Make your Diet Fit Your Specific Needs.

Cellular needs are different for each person based on their age, amount of activity, and health. Change the way you eat to meet these specific needs:

People who are active should focus on carbs and protein to help them heal and get energy. Adults over 50 should focus on vitamins and omega-3s to fight the loss of cells that comes with getting older. People with long-term illnesses should work with a doctor to figure out their unique dietary needs in order to improve the health of their cells.

To make a diet that supports cellular health, you need to make decisions that are high in nutrients, balanced in macronutrients, and low in harmful exposures. You can make a diet that supports healthy health at the cellular level by including foods that reduce inflammation, help you stay hydrated, and time your meals to fit your body's natural rhythms. Remember that every bite is a chance to feed your cells and make you healthier.

The Mediterranean Diet, Keto, and Plant-Based Options

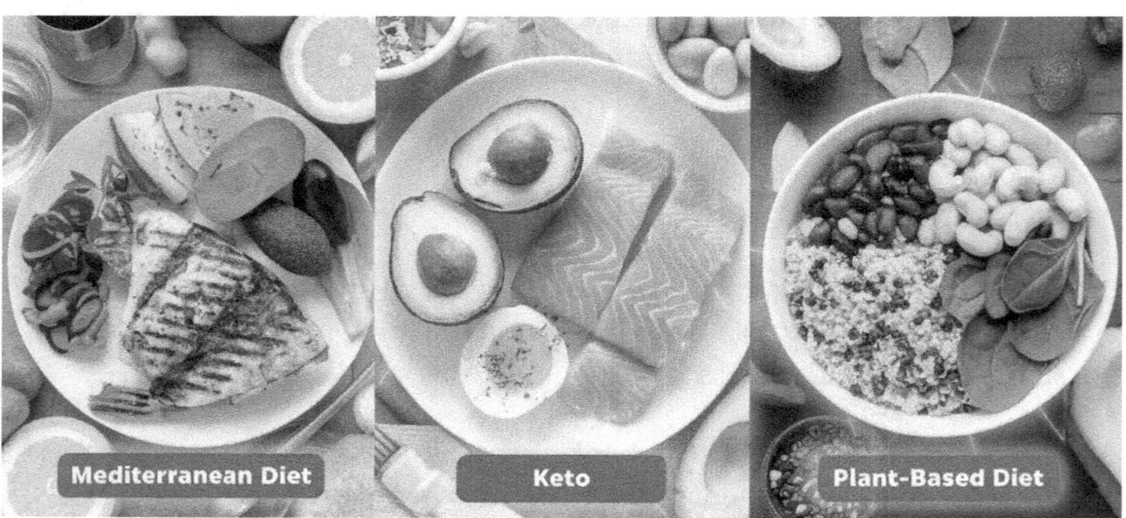

94

As you work to improve the health of your cells, each dietary plan has its own benefits. The Mediterranean diet, the ketogenic (keto) diet, and the plant-based diet are all different ways to feed cells and make them work better. Here is a more in-depth look at these foods and how they can help keep cells healthy.

The Mediterranean Diet

The Mediterranean diet is based on the traditional ways of eating in countries that are close to the Mediterranean Sea. People praise it for its high nutrient content and ability to reduce inflammation. It focuses on eating whole, barely processed foods that are high in fiber, healthy fats, and antioxidants. This makes it a beneficial choice for keeping cells healthy.

Important Parts of the Mediterranean Diet

Healthy fats primarily come from nuts, olive oil, and fatty fish.

Lean Proteins: The best sources are seafood and fish, but you should also eat chicken, eggs, and cheese in moderation.

Consume a variety of fruits and vegetables: they provide vitamins, minerals, and antioxidants that protect cells from oxidative stress.

Whole grains and legumes contain complex carbohydrates, which provide long-lasting energy, and fiber, which promotes gut health.

Herbs and spices: Instead of using too much salt, use natural herbs like oregano, basil, and turmeric, which are high in antioxidants.

Benefits for Cellular Health

Reduces inflammation: Omega-3 fatty acids found in fish and monounsaturated fatty acids found in olive oil lower inflammation and protect cell structures.

Fruits and vegetables that are high in antioxidants, such as tomatoes, spinach, and berries, fight free radicals that damage DNA and cell walls.

Better mitochondrial function: Whole grains and beans provide steady energy that helps cells make energy.

How to Implement the Mediterranean Diet

When cooking, use olive oil instead of butter. Eat fish like mackerel or salmon twice a week. Veggies should make up half of your plate at every meal. Instead of processed food, eat nuts, seeds, or fresh fruit as a snack.

The Ketogenic Food Plan

Cutting carbs and eating more fat is the ketogenic diet. The body enters a state known as ketosis as a result. During ketosis, the body gets most of its energy from ketones that come from fat instead of glucose. This change in metabolism affects the energy and healing of cells.

The Most Important Parts Of The Ketogenic Diet Are:

Eating a lot of fat; about 70–80% of your daily calories should come from healthy fats like avocados, coconut oil, and fatty foods.

Moderate protein: about 15 to 20 percent, coming from foods like tofu, eggs, and chicken.

Very Low Carbohydrates: Only 5–10% of daily calories should come from carbs, mostly from non-starchy veggies like zucchini and leafy greens.

Benefits for Cellular Health

Better mitochondrial efficiency: ketones are a cleaner source of energy than glucose, so metabolism makes fewer free radicals.

Helps autophagy: The keto diet can help autophagy, a process that cells use to get rid of broken parts and make cells work better.

Less reactive stress: Eating few carbohydrates keeps blood sugar levels stable, which lowers inflammation.

Considerations for Implementation

Cut back on carbs slowly to make getting into ketosis easier.

Choose healthy fats like nuts, seeds, and olive oil over processed fats.

Keep an eye on your electrolyte levels because the keto diet can cause changes that make it hard for cells to stay hydrated.

Possible Problems

The keto diet may not be right for everyone, even though it works for some. People with certain health problems or who are trying to eat more fiber may find it hard to stick to this eating plan.

Plant-Based Diets

People on a plant-based diet eat mostly foods that come from plants, like whole grains, nuts, seeds, legumes, fruits, and veggies. Depending on personal tastes and dietary goals, it either doesn't include animal goods or uses them very little.

Core Components of a Plant-Based Diet

Fruits and vegetables are the building blocks of a plant-based diet. They provide a wide range of enzymes, vitamins, and minerals.

Pulses and legumes are good sources of iron, fiber, and protein that come from plants.

Whole grains, like oats, brown rice, quinoa, and others, give you B vitamins and complex carbs.

Nuts and seeds: They have good fats and small amounts of nutrients like magnesium and zinc.

Benefits for Cellular Health

Foods that are high in plants have a lot of *antioxidants* like vitamins C and E, polyphenols, and pigments that keep cells safe from oxidative stress.

Fiber for detoxification: fiber improves gut health and helps get rid of toxins, which lowers inflammation in cells.

Less inflammation: the lack of animal fats and the presence of anti-inflammatory plant substances help keep cells healthy.

Plant-Based Diet Options

Vegetarian: Eggs and cheese are sources of protein and calcium.

Vegan: Doesn't eat any goods made from animals and gets their nutrients, like B12 and omega-3s, from fortified foods and different plants.

Flexitarian: Eating mostly plants but sometimes animal products, which gives you options while still supporting cell health.

How to Make the Switch to a Plant-Based Diet

Starting with "Meatless Mondays" or some other small promise can help. Use tofu, tempeh, or legumes instead of meat for nutrition. Eat a range of fruits, veggies, and grains to get a wide range of nutrients.

Comparing the Diets for Cellular Health

There are good things about each of these eating plans:

The Mediterranean Diet is very sustainable, full of substances that reduce inflammation and protect cells from damage, and helps cells stay healthy overall. The ketogenic diet supports autophagy and improves the function of mitochondria, making it a good choice for people with specific metabolic needs. Plant-based diets are great because they provide a lot of fiber and vitamins, which help the body get rid of toxins and reduce inflammation.

How to Pick the Best Diet

The best diet for each person relies on their health goals, personal tastes, and medical conditions.

For example: People who have chronic inflammation may benefit most from the Mediterranean or plant-based diets.

People who want to control their blood sugar or improve the function of their mitochondria may want to look into the keto diet.

In the end, mixing the best parts of these diets—for example, Mediterranean fats, intermittent fasting that works with ketosis, and a variety of plant-based foods—can offer a complete approach to cellular health.

Key Dietary Principles for Cellular Health

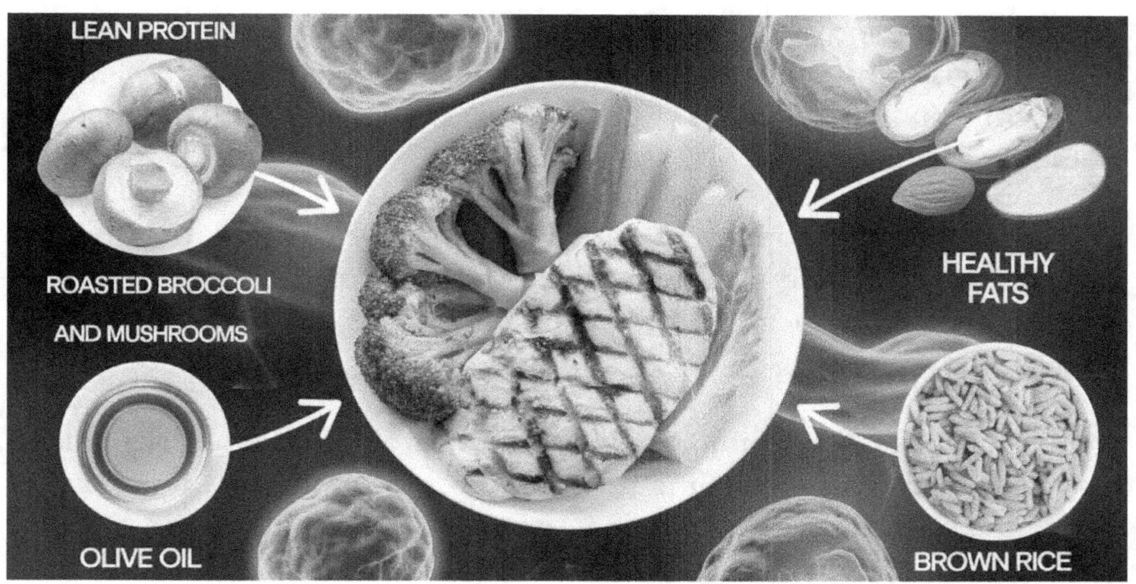

You must consciously choose nutrient-dense foods, ensure an even distribution of macronutrients, and lead a life that minimizes cellular stress in order to support cell health through eating. Here, we'll talk about the basic ideas behind a diet that is meant to feed and restore every cell in the body.

Put Whole, Unprocessed Foods First.

Foods that are in their original state are best for cells. Processed foods often lack fiber, vitamins, and minerals that our bodies need. They also contain high levels of sugar, unhealthy fats, and chemicals that harm our cells.

Why It Matters: Whole foods are full of vitamins, antioxidants, and bioavailable nutrients that keep cells safe from oxidative damage and help them work well.

What to Do: Pick fresh fruits and veggies over canned or frozen ones that have extra sugars or chemicals added to them. Try quinoa, brown rice, and oats instead of white bread or pasta if you want to eat whole carbs. Use nuts, seeds, or raw vegetables instead of boxed snacks.

Find the Right Balance Of Macronutrients For Cellular Efficiency.

Carbohydrates, proteins, and fats are the macronutrients that give cells energy, help them fix themselves, and keep them healthy. Finding the right mix makes cells work better and lessens the stress on metabolic processes.

Carbohydrates give you energy quickly, especially to cells that need a lot of it, like brain and muscle cells. Eat a lot of complex carbs, such as whole grains, legumes, and veggies, to ensure a steady release of glucose.

Proteins provide the amino acids cells need to fix themselves, make enzymes, and keep their immune systems strong. Eat a variety of foods, like eggs, dairy, nuts, beans, tofu, lean meats, and more.

Fats are necessary for cell walls to stay intact and for the body to make energy. Eat lots of avocados, olive oil, fatty fish, and seeds to get beneficial fats.

Ideal Ratios of Macronutrients

While individual needs vary, a general guideline is to consume 45–65% carbohydrates, with a focus on fiber-rich, whole-food sources. Depending on the age and level of activity, the protein content ranges from 10 to 35%. Fats range from 20 to 35 percent, with trans and heavy fats being the least important.

Eat a Range Of Foods That Are High In Micronutrients.

Micronutrients, like vitamins and minerals, help cells do many things, like making energy, fixing DNA, and protecting cells from damage.

Why it's important: Even small gaps can hurt the health of cells, making them tired, slow to heal, or more likely to be damaged by oxidative stress.

Things to pay attention to: Iron helps move oxygen around the body. You can find it in spinach, lentils, and lean foods. Nuts, seeds, and legumes contain zinc, which is beneficial for your immune system. Almonds, dark chocolate, and whole grains are all beneficial sources of magnesium, which helps your body use energy. Carrots, oranges, and nuts all have vitamins A, C, and E, which are antioxidants that protect cells.

Focus on Foods That Reduce Inflammation.

Long-term inflammation messes up the way cells work and makes diseases like cancer, diabetes, and heart problems more likely. An anti-inflammatory diet can lower the stress on cells and help them work at their best.

Important Foods: Fish high in fat, like salmon and mackerel, for omega-3 ins. Berries, citrus foods, and leafy greens are excellent sources of vitamin C and polyphenols. Turmeric and ginger because they contain substances that reduce inflammation.

Stay Hydrated To Make Cells Work Better.

Water is essential for keeping the balance of fluids, moving nutrients around, and getting rid of waste from cells. Dehydration can make it harder for cells to make energy and cause them to stop working properly.

Every day, we give you advice: At least 2–3 liters of water a day is a healthy goal, but it depends on how active you are and the weather.

Ways to keep drinking water: Consume foods rich in water content, such as oranges, cucumbers, and tomatoes. Limit beverages that dehydrate you, such as wine and coffee.

Watch How Much Sugar You Eat.

Cells can't handle too much sugar, which can cause oxidative stress and inflammation. Cutting down on extra sugars helps keep blood sugar levels steady and eases the strain on the metabolism.

Why it's important: Glycation happens faster when you eat a lot of sugar. Sugar accelerates this damage to proteins and cell function.

What to do: Eat fresh fruits instead of sugary snacks. Avoid using excessive amounts of honey, stevia, or other natural sugars. Avoid consuming sweet drinks such as energy drinks and sodas.

Eat Foods That Are High In Phytonutrients And Antioxidants.

Antioxidants eliminate free radicals, thereby preventing oxidative damage to cell structures. Plants contain phytonutrients, which fortify cells against disease and aging.

Important Sources: Some foods that are beneficial for you are dark leafy greens, bright vegetables, and fruits. Green tea's catechins shield DNA from free radical damage. For antioxidants, opt for dark chocolate that contains at least 70% cocoa.

Keep Your Gut Healthy

The gut microbiome is an important part of cellular health because it helps with digestion, makes some vitamins, and controls inflammation. A healthy gut microbiome makes it easier for the body to absorb nutrients and get rid of toxins.

Things to Put In: Yogurt, kefir, and fermented foods like cabbage and kimchi contain probiotics, which are beneficial for your health. Prebiotics are beneficial bacteria found in foods such as garlic, onions, bananas, and asparagus.

Limit Exposure to Toxins and Pollutants

Consuming fewer pollutants reduces cell load and speeds detoxification.

What to Do: To avoid chemicals, choose organic food when you can. Limit processed meats because they often have dangerous preservatives in them, like nitrates. Do not use metal or non-stick pans for cooking because they give off chemicals that are harmful for you.

Stick to the Same Meal Times Every Day.

Setting up regular eating habits helps keep circadian rhythms in check and supports metabolic processes at the cellular level. By increasing autophagy and lowering reactive stress, intermittent fasting or eating only at certain times can also be helpful.

By following these tips every day, you can build an eating pattern that supports and improves the health of your cells, laying the groundwork for long-term vitality and resilience.

How to Build Balanced, Nutrient-Rich Meals

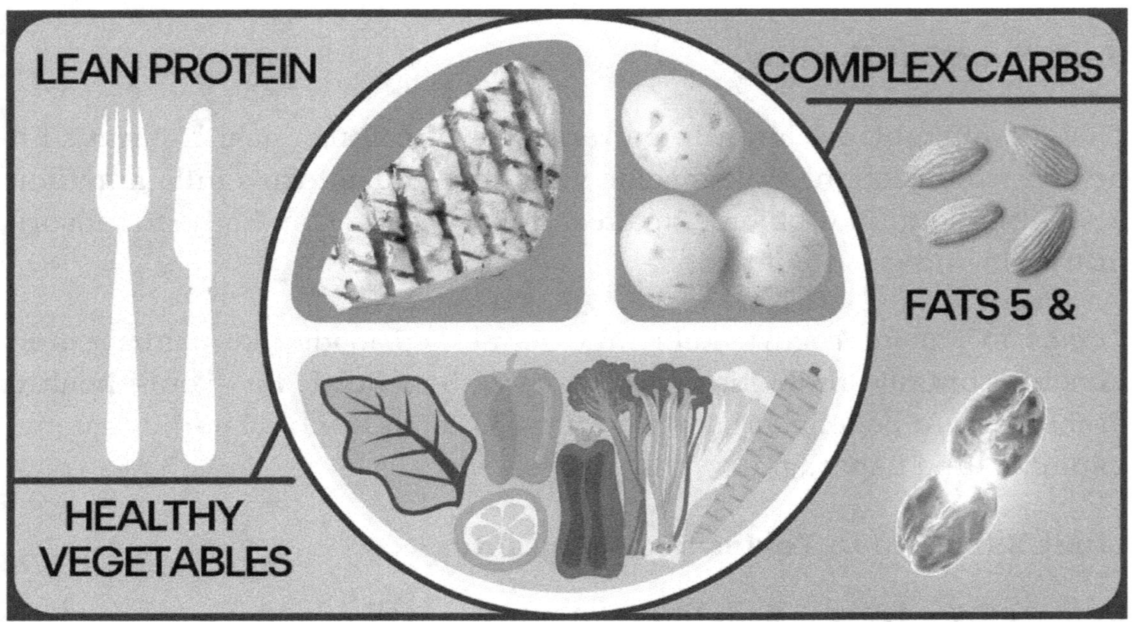

Making meals that are well-balanced and full of nutrients is important for keeping cells healthy and for your general health. A well-planned meal contains the right mix of macronutrients, micronutrients, and antioxidants. These are essential for generating energy, repairing cells, and combating oxidative stress. Here is a full guide to help you make meals that are beneficial for your cells.

Begin with the Plate Method.

The plate method is a simple but useful way to plan meals that are both visually appealing and full of nutrients. Here's how to divide your plate:

50% Fruits and Vegetables: Choose a range of colors to get the most phytonutrients and antioxidants.

25% Lean Protein: Find amino acids from both plant and animal sources.

25% whole grains or starchy vegetables: These give you long-lasting energy through complex carbs.

An example of a meal: On the side, there are roasted broccoli, carrots, and red peppers. For protein, eat beans or grilled chicken breast. Quinoa or sweet potatoes for carbs.

Use a Wide Range of Colors.

Eating a wide variety of brightly colored fruits and veggies is the best way to get a wide range of antioxidants, vitamins, and minerals. Each color stands for a different phytonutrient that is beneficial for cell health in its own way.

Red: Tomatoes, strawberries, and red peppers are excellent sources of lycopene and anthocyanins, which protect against oxidative stress.

Orange and yellow (beta-carotene and vitamin C): As a group, carrots, oranges, and squash are good for your skin and immune system.

Green (Chlorophyll, Folate): Spinach, kale, and bananas help the body get rid of toxins and fix DNA.

Blue and purple (anthocyanins and resveratrol): Blueberries, eggplants, and purple cabbage are good for your heart and brain.

White or brown (allicin, selenium): Onions, garlic, and mushrooms help the thyroid and immune system work.

Balance Macronutrients in Every Meal

Each macronutrient is important for cell health in its own way, and eating all three makes sure that your meals give you long-lasting energy and fullness.

Carbohydrates: Eat complex carbs like beans, chickpeas, brown rice, oats, and other whole grains. Also eat starchy veggies like sweet potatoes and squash. Eat fewer processed carbs and artificial sugars, which raise blood sugar and make inflammation worse.

Proteins: Choose lean meats like chicken, fish, and turkey, or plant-based proteins like tofu, tempeh, rice, and beans. Eat a complete protein with every meal to get the necessary amino acids your body needs to repair cells and make enzymes.

Fats: Pay attention to good fats that come from foods like bananas, nuts, seeds, olive oil, and fatty fish. Stay away from prepared foods that are high in trans fats and saturated fats.

Eat Foods That Are High In Fiber.

Fiber is important for cleansing, keeping blood sugar in check, and gut health. Try to eat foods that have both soluble and insoluble fiber.

Soluble fiber is found in flaxseeds, oats, and apples. It helps lower cholesterol and keep blood sugar stable.

Insoluble fiber: This type of fiber is found in nuts, veggies, and whole grains and helps the body digest food and get rid of waste.

Add a Good Amount of Antioxidants.

Antioxidants slow down the aging process and protect cells from damage caused by free radicals. At every meal, eat something that is high in vitamins.

For example, put some blueberries on your food. Add a dressing made with green tea or matcha. Add turmeric or cinnamon to food to make it healthier and more antioxidant-rich.

Use Healthy Cooking Methods

The nutrients and health effects of food can change depending on how you cook it. Choose ways to cook that keep nutrients and reduce harmful chemicals.

Steaming, baking, cooking, grilling, and stir-frying are the best ways to cook it.

Things to stay away from: charring and deep-frying, which make trans fats and free radicals that are bad for you.

Plan for Portion Control

When you eat too much, even healthy foods, your cells can't handle the extra calories and nutrients. Match your exercise level and metabolic needs to the right amount of food.

Tip: To avoid eating too much, use smaller plates. Pre-measure snacks so you don't eat without thinking. Pay attention to signs that you are hungry or full.

Don't forget to Drink Water.

Adding water-rich foods to your meals, like melons, cucumbers, and fresh greens, can help your cells stay hydrated in addition to drinking enough water.

Hydration Boosters: For a cool drink, add slices of lemon or cucumber to water. Soups and smoothies can also help you meet your daily fluid needs.

Include fermented Foods to keep your Gut Healthy.

It is important for cells to have a good gut microbiome because it improves the absorption of nutrients and lowers inflammation. Eat some cultured foods every day. Yogurt, kefir, cabbage, kimchi, miso, and kombucha are all examples.

Spice Up for Cellular Protection

Herbs and spices like ginger, cinnamon, mustard, and garlic can help your cells stay healthy by reducing inflammation and protecting cells from damage.

Turmeric: For the curcumin it contains, add it to smoothies, soups, or stews.

Garlic: For the most allicin release, mince raw garlic.

Ginger: To reduce swelling, add it to drinks or marinades.

Mind the Meal Timing

It's not always about what you eat, but when you eat. If you want your cells to work at their best, don't skip meals because it can throw off your blood sugar. Eat several small meals spread out throughout the day to keep your energy level steady. If you want to give your cells a break from digestion and boost autophagy, try eating only at certain times.

Meal Plans with Lots of Nutrients

Breakfast:

- *Greek yogurt topped with chia seeds, walnuts, and mixed berries (antioxidants, protein, omega-3s).*

- *A slice of whole-grain toast with avocado and a sprinkle of hemp seeds (fiber, healthy fats).*

Lunch:

- *Grilled salmon with quinoa and steamed broccoli (protein, complex carbs, vitamins).*

- *Side salad with spinach, cherry tomatoes, olive oil, and balsamic vinegar (phytonutrients, healthy fats).*

Dinner:

- *Stir-fried tofu with brown rice and a medley of bell peppers, onions, and zucchini (protein, carbs, antioxidants).*

- *Season with garlic, turmeric, and ginger for added health benefits.*

Snack Options:

- *A handful of almonds or mixed nuts.*

- *Hummus with carrot and cucumber sticks.*

- *Fresh fruit with a dollop of almond butter.*

By making meals that are high in nutrients and varied on a regular basis, you can properly fuel your body, improve the function of cells, and support long-term health.

CHAPTER 7

MONTHLY MEAL PLAN FOR CELLULAR HEALTH

A Quick Look at the Plan: Nutrient-Dense Meals That Give You Energy

The Monthly Meal Plan for Cellular Health focuses on meals that are high in nutrients and give you energy to help your cells work at their best. This plan meticulously designs each of the four weeks to concentrate on a distinct aspect of cellular health. The weeks go in order of building a strong foundation, detoxifying and repairing, reducing inflammation, and revitalizing. We carefully plan every meal to provide you with the vitamins, minerals, antioxidants, healthy fats, and other nutrients your cells require to stay healthy, repair themselves, and grow.

The plan operates on the following principles:

- *Whole, unprocessed foods:* Eating fewer processed foods lowers your risk of getting toxins and chemicals that are harmful for you.
- *Antioxidant-rich ingredients* protect cells from damage from oxidative stress and free radicals.
- *Healthy fats:* Cell walls and energy production can't happen without them.
- *High-quality protein* is essential for both healing and growth.
- *Fruits and veggies that are high in phytonutrients* help the body get rid of toxins and reduce inflammation.

By following this plan, you will not only feed your cells, but you will also have more energy, clearer thinking, better nutrition, and other long-term health benefits.

Week 1: Building Cellular Foundations

Setting the stage for ideal cellular health is the main focus of the first week of the monthly meal plan. During this time, your body gets the nutrients it needs for strong cell function. You can stay healthy for a long time by focusing on nutrient-dense foods that help your body make energy, fix cells, and keep membranes intact.

Goals for Week 1

1. *Help mitochondria work better:* Give your cells the nutrients they need to make more ATP to improve their energy sources.
2. *Support Cell Membrane Integrity:* To make cell membranes strong and flexible, eat healthy fats and proteins.
3. *Support antioxidant defense:* Eat foods that are high in antioxidants to lower reactive stress and keep cell structures safe.
4. *Hydration for Cellular Efficiency:* Ensure adequate hydration to facilitate the movement of nutrients and elimination of waste.

Important Nutrients for Building Blocks of Cells

Proteins: Building blocks of life, proteins enable cells to repair and regenerate. Adding high-quality protein to food helps keep cells and organs' structures strong. Eggs, turkey, tofu, tempeh, beans, fish, and low-fat dairy are all nutritious sources.

Healthy Fats: Healthy fats are important for making the lipid bilayer that keeps cell membranes flexible and helps nutrients move through them easily. Nuts, seeds (such as chia, flax, and pumpkin), avocados, and olive oil are all good sources.

Complex Carbohydrates: Complex carbs are a source of glucose that releases slowly, keeping energy levels steady and supporting cell activity. Oats, brown rice, quinoa, sweet potatoes, and whole-grain bread are all good sources.

Vitamins and Minerals: Vitamin B Complex: Helps the mitochondria work and the production of energy. You can find it in leafy veggies, eggs, and whole grains. Magnesium is needed for enzyme processes that make ATP. It's in spinach, nuts, and seeds. Iron promotes the flow of air to cells so they can make energy. It can be found in spinach, beans, and lean red meat.

Hydration: Staying properly hydrated helps cells do things like get rid of trash and absorb nutrients. Aim to drink at least two to three liters of water every day, and eat foods that are high in water, like watermelons and veggies.

Daily Meal Plan for Week 1

Day 1

Breakfast:

- Avocado toast on whole-grain bread with a poached egg.

- A side of mixed berries (blueberries, strawberries, and raspberries).

Mid-Morning Snack:

- A handful of raw almonds and a small apple.

Lunch:

- Grilled chicken salad with mixed greens, cherry tomatoes, cucumber, and a lemon-olive oil vinaigrette.

- A serving of quinoa on the side.

Afternoon Snack:

- Low-fat Greek yogurt topped with chia seeds and sliced banana.

Dinner:

- Baked salmon with roasted sweet potatoes and steamed broccoli.

- A small side of spinach sautéed in olive oil.

Evening Snack:

- Herbal tea with a square of dark chocolate (70% cocoa or higher).

Day 2

Breakfast:

- Spinach and mushroom omelet cooked in olive oil.

- A slice of whole-grain toast.

- A glass of unsweetened green tea.

Mid-Morning Snack:

- Carrot sticks with a tablespoon of hummus.

Lunch:

- Lentil and vegetable soup with a side of whole-grain crackers.

- Mixed greens topped with sunflower seeds and a lemon-tahini dressing.

Afternoon Snack:

- A handful of walnuts and a slice of pear.

Dinner:

- Grilled turkey breast with roasted Brussels sprouts and mashed cauliflower.

- A side of steamed green beans drizzled with olive oil.

Evening Snack:

- Chamomile tea with fresh kiwi slices.

Day 3

Breakfast:

- Steel-cut oatmeal topped with sliced almonds, fresh strawberries, and a drizzle of honey.

- A glass of almond milk.

Mid-Morning Snack:

- Celery sticks with almond butter.

Lunch:

- Tuna salad made with olive oil, lemon juice, celery, and parsley.

- A small baked sweet potato.

- Steamed asparagus on the side.

Afternoon Snack:

- Low-fat cottage cheese with pineapple chunks.

Dinner:

- Herb-roasted chicken thighs with quinoa and roasted zucchini.

- A side of kale sautéed with garlic.

Evening Snack:

- Peppermint tea with a few slices of orange.

Day 4

Breakfast:

- Smoothie made with spinach, frozen mango, almond milk, and a scoop of protein powder.

- A slice of whole-grain toast.

Mid-Morning Snack:

- A boiled egg and a handful of cherry tomatoes.

Lunch:

- Grilled shrimp with a wild rice pilaf and roasted bell peppers.

- A side salad with arugula and lemon dressing.

Afternoon Snack:

- A small handful of mixed nuts (walnuts, pecans, cashews).

Dinner:

- Pan-seared tofu with stir-fried broccoli, mushrooms, and carrots in a tamari-ginger sauce.

- A side of steamed edamame.

Evening Snack:

- A warm glass of almond milk with a pinch of cinnamon.

Day 5

Breakfast:

- Scrambled eggs with spinach, onions, and tomatoes.

- A slice of whole-grain bread.

- A glass of orange juice.

Mid-Morning Snack:

- Sliced cucumbers with guacamole.

Lunch:

- Grilled salmon over a bed of arugula, avocado, and grapefruit segments.

- A serving of barley on the side.

Afternoon Snack:

- A small serving of unsweetened trail mix with dried cranberries.

Dinner:

- Roast lamb chops with mashed sweet potatoes and steamed green beans.

- A side of roasted Brussels sprouts.

Evening Snack:

- Ginger tea with a square of dark chocolate.

Day 6

Breakfast:

- Whole-grain toast with almond butter and banana slices.

- A cup of black coffee or green tea.

Mid-Morning Snack:

- A hard-boiled egg and a handful of grapes.

Lunch:

- Grilled vegetable wrap with hummus in a whole-grain tortilla.

- A side of lentil soup.

Afternoon Snack:

- A small smoothie made with unsweetened yogurt, frozen berries, and spinach.

Dinner:

- Baked cod with roasted cauliflower and a side of wild rice.

- Steamed carrots drizzled with a touch of olive oil.

Evening Snack:

- Herbal tea with fresh apple slices.

Day 7

Breakfast:

- Chia pudding made with almond milk, topped with fresh blueberries and a sprinkle of shredded coconut.

- A cup of green tea.

Mid-Morning Snack:

- Sliced bell peppers with a tablespoon of tzatziki.

Lunch:

- Grilled chicken breast with a quinoa and roasted vegetable medley (zucchini, red onion, eggplant).

- A side of baby spinach drizzled with balsamic vinegar.

Afternoon Snack:

- Greek yogurt with walnuts and a drizzle of honey.

Dinner:

- Pan-seared salmon with sautéed kale and garlic.

- A serving of roasted butternut squash.

Evening Snack:

- Warm chamomile tea with a small piece of pear.

Highlights of the Shopping List

Proteins: Eggs, chicken, turkey, salmon, cod, shrimp, tofu, beans, Greek yogurt, and cottage cheese are all excellent sources of protein.

Fats: Avocado, olive oil, nuts (almonds, walnuts), and seeds (chia, flax, sunflower) are all beneficial sources of fat.

Carbohydrates: Quinoa, sweet potatoes, brown rice, oats, and whole-grain bread are all beneficial sources of carbs.

Vegetables: Spinach, broccoli, kale, asparagus, zucchini, Brussels sprouts, carrots, bell peppers, and spinach.

Fruits: pineapple, berries, bananas, oranges, kiwis, grapes, and oranges.

Other options: Includes almond milk, herbal teas, and dark chocolate that contains 70% or more cocoa.

This plan makes sure that your meals are varied and full of nutrients, which is beneficial for your cells and keeps you interested and enjoying the week.

Meal Preparation Tips

1. *Batch cooking:* To save time, make a lot of grilled chicken, tofu, lentils, and carbs (like quinoa or brown rice) at the beginning of the week.
2. *Make snacks:* Put nuts, seeds, and fruits in packages that you can grab and go.
3. *Don't forget to drink water.* Always have a bottle on hand, and for taste, add cucumber or lemon slices.

Benefits of Week 1 Focus

1. *More energy:* This week's work on improving mitochondrial activity gives you energy that lasts all day.

2. *Health of the Cell Membrane:* Good fats make cells stronger, so they can resist damage and better share nutrients.
3. *Better antioxidant defense:* Foods high in antioxidants lower reactive stress, which helps cells work properly over time.
4. *Getting the nutrients you need:* Eating well-balanced meals makes sure your cells get the minerals and vitamins they need to grow.

Lifestyle Tips for Cellular Support During Week 1

1. Physical Activity: To spark mitochondrial activity, do light exercises like yoga, walks, or strength training.
2. Enough Sleep: Aim for 7 to 9 hours of adequate sleep each night to let your cells heal and grow back.
3. Dealing with stress: Mindfulness or meditation can help lower cortisol levels, which can hurt the health of cells.

By following the plan for Week 1, you'll build a strong base for your cells that gets your body ready for Week 2's focus on cleansing and repair. This methodical approach ensures the nourishment, stimulation, and optimal performance of your cells.

Week 2: Detox and Repair

Through the second week of the Monthly Meal Plan for Cellular Health, you will be focusing on cleaning out your body and fixing damaged cells. This step equips your body with tools to eliminate toxins, reduce oxidative stress, and repair damaged cells. The meals are light but full of nutrients. They are high in antioxidants, fiber, and vitamins that help the liver, kidneys, and skin clean out the body.

Goals for Week 2

1. Get rid of toxins: Eat foods that are beneficial for the liver, like cruciferous veggies, lemon, and turmeric, to help the body's natural detox pathways.

2. Help cells heal: eat foods that are high in antioxidants, amino acids, and important fatty acids to help cells heal and grow again.
3. Improve Gut Health: Eat fermentation and fiber-rich foods to make your gut work better, since the gut is an important part of getting rid of toxins.
4. Hydrate: Drink more water to get rid of toxins and keep your cells moist. For variety, add herbal drinks or water with herbs in it.

Key Foods for Detox and Repair

1. *Cruciferous Vegetables:* Broccoli, cauliflower, kale, Brussels sprouts, and cabbage are rich in glucosinolates, which aid the liver's enzymes in eliminating toxins.
2. *Citrus fruits:* Oranges, lemons, and limes raise glutathione levels and give you vitamin C, which helps your body heal itself.
3. *Beets:* Beets are full of betaine and nitrates, which help the liver work better and give cells more air.
4. *Garlic and onions:* They have sulfur molecules that help the body get rid of toxins.
5. *Spices and herbs:* Turmeric, ginger, cilantro, and parsley can help lower swelling and get rid of heavy metals.
6. *Green Tea:* Green tea fights free radicals and is beneficial for the liver because it has a lot of catechins.
7. *Fermented foods:* Kimchi, cabbage, kefir, and yogurt all have probiotics that help keep the bacteria in your gut in balance.
8. *Omega-3s:* Flaxseeds, salmon, and walnuts contain these. They help repair cell membranes and lower inflammation.
9. *Hydration boosters:* Coconut water, cucumber, and watermelon all help the body get rid of toxins and replace minerals.

Daily Meal Plan for Week 2

Day 1

- **Breakfast**: Warm lemon water followed by an avocado smoothie (spinach, cucumber, lemon, and almond milk).

- **Snack**: Fresh carrot and celery sticks with hummus.

- **Lunch**: Detox salad with kale, roasted beets, avocado, quinoa, and a turmeric-lemon vinaigrette.

- **Snack**: A handful of raw almonds and a cup of green tea.

- **Dinner**: Baked cod with steamed broccoli, roasted cauliflower, and a side of mashed sweet potatoes.

- **Evening Drink**: Chamomile tea with grated ginger.

Day 2

- **Breakfast**: Chia seed pudding made with almond milk, topped with blueberries and shredded coconut.

- **Snack**: Sliced cucumber and a green apple.

- **Lunch**: Lentil and vegetable stew with a side of whole-grain bread.

- **Snack**: Greek yogurt with a sprinkle of flaxseeds.

- **Dinner**: Grilled salmon with sautéed spinach and roasted carrots.

- **Evening Drink**: Warm water with a slice of lemon.

Day 3

- **Breakfast**: Smoothie bowl with frozen mango, spinach, and unsweetened yogurt, topped with pumpkin seeds and pomegranate arils.

- **Snack**: A boiled egg and a handful of walnuts.

- **Lunch**: Brown rice with stir-fried tofu, broccoli, and sesame seeds.

- **Snack**: A pear and a few slices of avocado.

- **Dinner**: Herb-roasted chicken breast with a side of steamed asparagus and mashed cauliflower.

- **Evening Drink**: Ginger and mint tea.

Day 4

- **Breakfast**: Scrambled eggs with sautéed mushrooms and spinach, served with a slice of whole-grain toast.

- **Snack**: Orange slices with a few raw cashews.

- **Lunch**: Detox Buddha bowl with quinoa, chickpeas, kale, roasted sweet potatoes, and tahini dressing.

- **Snack**: A cup of kefir with fresh berries.

- **Dinner**: Baked trout with zucchini noodles and roasted Brussels sprouts.

- **Evening Drink**: Hibiscus tea with a teaspoon of honey.

Day 5

- **Breakfast**: Steel-cut oats with a drizzle of honey, chia seeds, and diced pear.

- **Snack**: Sliced red bell pepper with guacamole.

- **Lunch**: Spinach and lentil curry served with brown rice.

- **Snack**: A small handful of mixed nuts and dried cranberries.

- **Dinner**: Grilled shrimp with a citrus salad (arugula, grapefruit, avocado) and a side of roasted beets.

- **Evening Drink**: Green tea with lemon.

Day 6

- **Breakfast**: Matcha smoothie with banana, spinach, almond milk, and a tablespoon of chia seeds.

- **Snack**: A boiled egg and a small handful of almonds.

- **Lunch**: Tomato and cucumber quinoa salad with grilled chicken and a drizzle of olive oil.

- **Snack**: Greek yogurt with a sprinkle of sunflower seeds.

- **Dinner**: Pan-seared tofu with stir-fried bok choy and steamed brown rice.

- **Evening Drink**: Warm water infused with cucumber and mint.

Day 7

- **Breakfast**: Smoothie bowl with frozen berries, unsweetened almond milk, and spinach, topped with shredded coconut and chia seeds.

- **Snack**: Sliced pear with almond butter.

- **Lunch**: Wild rice with roasted salmon and a side of steamed broccoli and lemon dressing.

- **Snack**: A small serving of trail mix (walnuts, pumpkin seeds, dried apricots).

- **Dinner**: Lentil soup with a side of sautéed kale and whole-grain toast.

- **Evening Drink**: Herbal tea with fresh ginger slices.

Week 3: Anti-Inflammatory and Anti-Aging Meals

The third week of the Cellular Health Diet is all about lowering inflammation and helping cells live longer. Chronic inflammation exacerbates damage to cells, aging, and illnesses such as diabetes, heart disease, and neurodegenerative disorders. The foods on this week's plan are high in nutrients, fight inflammation, and protect cells from damage. It's like slowing down the aging process at the molecular level.

Goals for Week 3

1. *Lower inflammation:* Eat foods that are high in polyphenols, omega-3 fatty acids, and natural substances that reduce inflammation.

2. Make cells live longer: Eat foods that are high in nutrients to help your body make telomerase, an enzyme that guards the ends of DNA strands (called telomeres).

3. *Increase your intake of antioxidants:* Provide your body with a variety of antioxidants to combat free radicals and prevent reactive stress.

4. *Support Skin and Joint Health:* For healthy skin, hair, and joints, eat foods that boost collagen and keep you hydrated.

Key Foods that Fight Inflammation and Slow Down Aging

1. *Fruits and vegetables:* Berries (like blueberries, strawberries, and raspberries): These are high in flavonoids and anthocyanins, which fight inflammation.
   Leafy greens like spinach, kale, and Swiss chard are high in vitamins A, C, and E, which help cells heal.
   Cruciferous vegetables, such as broccoli and Brussels sprouts, contain sulforaphane, an anti-inflammatory chemical.
   Avocado is full of beneficial fats, vitamins, and antioxidants.

2. *Healthy Fats:* Flaxseeds, chia seeds, walnuts, and fatty fish like salmon and mackerel contain omega-3s, which fight inflammation.
   Olive oil is an important part of anti-inflammatory foods like the Mediterranean diet.

3. *Whole Grains:* Quinoa, oats, and brown rice all have fiber, which is beneficial for your gut health and reduces inflammation.

4. *Spices and herbs:* Turmeric mixed with black pepper is a powerful pain reliever. Ginger: It reduces swelling and improves digestion. Rosemary and thyme are full of polyphenols that fight age.

5. *Eat nuts and seeds.* Pumpkin seeds, almonds, walnuts, and sunflower seeds are all beneficial for you because they have iron and vitamin E.

6. *Foods High in Probiotics:* Fermented foods such as kefir, sauerkraut, and miso enhance the health of your gut bacteria, a direct correlation to reduced inflammation.

7. *Herbal and green teas* are high in catechins, which lower inflammation and oxidative stress.

8. *Foods that keep you hydrated:* Cucumbers, strawberries, and bone broth keep your skin flexible and your joints smooth.

Daily Meal Plan for Week 3

Day 1

- **Breakfast**: Greek yogurt with blueberries, chia seeds, and a drizzle of honey.

- **Snack**: A handful of walnuts and a green tea.

- **Lunch**: Grilled salmon with a quinoa and spinach salad, topped with olive oil and lemon dressing.

- **Snack**: Cucumber slices with hummus.

- **Dinner**: Turmeric-spiced lentil soup with a side of roasted broccoli and sweet potatoes.

- **Evening Drink**: Chamomile tea with a slice of ginger.

Day 2

- **Breakfast**: Avocado toast on whole-grain bread, topped with a poached egg and fresh parsley.

- **Snack**: A sliced apple with almond butter.

- **Lunch**: Mediterranean chickpea salad with cucumbers, tomatoes, olives, and a tahini-lemon dressing.

- **Snack**: A small handful of dark chocolate (70% cocoa) and green tea.

- **Dinner**: Grilled mackerel with steamed kale and a wild rice pilaf.

- **Evening Drink**: Hibiscus tea with honey.

Day 3

- **Breakfast**: Smoothie made with spinach, frozen berries, almond milk, and flaxseeds.

- **Snack**: A boiled egg and a handful of mixed nuts.

- **Lunch**: Brown rice bowl with stir-fried tofu, broccoli, and ginger sesame dressing.

- **Snack**: Fresh orange slices with a sprinkle of cinnamon.

- **Dinner**: Baked chicken breast with turmeric-spiced cauliflower and roasted carrots.

- **Evening Drink**: Warm water with lemon.

Day 4

- **Breakfast**: Steel-cut oats with sliced banana, a sprinkle of cinnamon, and crushed pecans.

- **Snack**: Greek yogurt with a drizzle of honey and sunflower seeds.

- **Lunch**: Herb-roasted turkey breast with a mixed greens salad and balsamic vinaigrette.

- **Snack**: A small serving of sauerkraut and cucumber slices.

- **Dinner**: Baked cod with a side of zucchini noodles and a kale-pomegranate salad.

- **Evening Drink**: Ginger and turmeric tea.

Day 5

- **Breakfast**: Chia pudding made with almond milk, topped with kiwi slices and shredded coconut.

- **Snack**: A handful of almonds and green tea.

- **Lunch**: Lentil and vegetable curry with a side of steamed brown rice.

- **Snack**: Fresh strawberries with a dollop of unsweetened yogurt.

- **Dinner**: Grilled shrimp with an avocado and grapefruit salad.

- **Evening Drink**: Peppermint tea.

Day 6

- **Breakfast**: Omelet with spinach, mushrooms, and turmeric, served with whole-grain toast.

- **Snack**: A pear with a few walnuts.

- **Lunch**: Wild rice salad with roasted sweet potatoes, chickpeas, and tahini dressing.

- **Snack**: Sliced carrots and celery with guacamole.

- **Dinner**: Herb-roasted lamb with a side of Brussels sprouts and mashed parsnips.

- **Evening Drink**: Chamomile tea with a pinch of cinnamon.

Day 7

- **Breakfast**: Smoothie bowl with frozen mango, spinach, and almond milk, topped with pumpkin seeds and cacao nibs.

- **Snack**: A boiled egg and a few cashews.

- **Lunch**: Roasted salmon with a quinoa and arugula salad, drizzled with olive oil and lemon.

- **Snack**: Sliced bell peppers with a yogurt-based dip.

- **Dinner**: Ginger-garlic chicken stir-fry with bok choy and wild rice.

- **Evening Drink**: Herbal tea with fresh mint leaves.

Additional Tips for Anti-Inflammatory and Anti-Aging Success

1. *Use colorful plates.* Brightly colored fruits and vegetables are rich in antioxidants.
2. *Put healthy fats first.* Omega-3s are crucial for brain health and lowering inflammation.
3. *Eat less of foods that make inflammation worse.* Stay away from processed sugars, fried foods, and refined carbs.
4. *Use a lot of spices.* You should always have turmeric, cinnamon, and ginger on hand when you cook.
5. *Stay hydrated:* To keep your cells working properly and your skin's flexibility, drink water regularly and eat foods that are high in water.
6. *Practice mindful eating.* Eating slowly and deliberately helps your body digest food and absorb nutrients.

By following this plan to fight inflammation and slow down aging, you give your body the tools it needs to fight inflammation, protect cells from damage, and make you live longer overall.

Week 4: Revitalization and Energy Boosting

During the last week of the Cellular Health Diet, the focus is on recharging energy stores, speeding up the metabolism, and giving the body foods that help cells heal and stay healthy. Because you went through the foundational, detoxifying, and anti-inflammatory phases, your body is better able to keep its cells healthy by the end of this trip. Week 4 builds upon this progress by emphasizing foods that restore vitality, maintain high energy levels, and enhance general health.

Goals for Week 4

1. *Refill Nutrient Stores:* Replace the essential nutrients lost as a result of stress, the environment, and detoxification.
2. *Boost Cellular Energy:* Foods that are high in nutrients and energy can help your body make more ATP, which is the energy currency of cells.
3. *Help the mitochondria work properly* by giving them foods that improve their health; mitochondria are the powerhouses of cells.
4. *To live longer,* focus on nutrients that slow down aging and adaptogens that keep your energy and vigor high over time.
5. *Keep your cellular health* at its best by keeping your blood sugar levels steady, taking care of your gut, and lowering oxidative stress.

Key Nutrients for Rejuvenation and Energy Boosting

1. *Complex Carbohydrates:* Whole grains, sweet potatoes, and beans keep blood sugar levels steady, which gives you long-lasting energy.
2. *Lean Proteins:* Plant-based proteins like tofu, tempeh, lentils, and chicken, fish, and eggs fix cell structures and help the body heal.
3. *Good fats:* Omega-3s from fish and nuts are beneficial for your heart and brain, and medium-chain triglycerides (MCTs) from coconut oil give you energy right away.
4. *B-Vitamins:* Whole grains, eggs, and leafy vegetables contain these vitamins. They are essential for the nervous system and energy metabolism.

5. Foods like spinach, quinoa, pumpkin seeds, and beans contain minerals like *iron and magnesium.* The body needs them to transport air and produce energy.
6. *Adaptogens:* Herbs like ginseng, ashwagandha, and rhodiola help fight stress and make you stronger.
7. *Probiotics and prebiotics:* Consuming fermented foods such as kimchi, kefir, and yogurt, along with prebiotic-rich foods like onions, bananas, and garlic, contributes to maintaining a healthy gut and boosting energy levels.
8. *Staying hydrated:* Fruits that are high in water, like tomatoes and oranges, and drinks that are high in electrolytes can help you keep your energy and fluid balance.

Daily Meal Plan for Week 4

Day 1

- **Breakfast**: Oatmeal topped with sliced banana, walnuts, and a drizzle of honey.

- **Snack**: A handful of almonds and a green tea with lemon.

- **Lunch**: Grilled chicken breast with a quinoa and arugula salad, dressed with olive oil and balsamic vinegar.

- **Snack**: Carrot sticks with guacamole.

- **Dinner**: Baked salmon with roasted Brussels sprouts and sweet potatoes.

- **Evening Drink**: Warm water with a splash of apple cider vinegar.

Day 2

- **Breakfast**: Greek yogurt with mixed berries, chia seeds, and shredded coconut.

- **Snack**: Sliced apple with almond butter.

- **Lunch**: Lentil soup with a side of whole-grain toast.

- **Snack**: A small handful of dark chocolate (70% cocoa) and green tea.

- **Dinner**: Stir-fried tofu with bok choy, mushrooms, and wild rice.

- **Evening Drink**: Chamomile tea.

Day 3

- **Breakfast**: Smoothie made with spinach, pineapple, coconut water, and a scoop of protein powder.

- **Snack**: Hard-boiled egg with a few cherry tomatoes.

- **Lunch**: Herb-roasted turkey slices with a kale-pomegranate salad.

- **Snack**: Cucumber slices with hummus.

- **Dinner**: Grilled cod with zucchini noodles and roasted carrots.

- **Evening Drink**: Mint tea.

Day 4

- **Breakfast**: Scrambled eggs with sautéed spinach and mushrooms, served with whole-grain toast.

- **Snack**: A handful of trail mix with dried cranberries, almonds, and sunflower seeds.

- **Lunch**: Brown rice bowl with black beans, roasted red peppers, and avocado slices.

- **Snack**: Sliced pear with a sprinkle of cinnamon.

- **Dinner**: Baked chicken thighs with turmeric-spiced cauliflower and steamed green beans.

- **Evening Drink**: Ginger tea.

Day 5

- **Breakfast**: Chia pudding made with almond milk, topped with mango chunks and pumpkin seeds.

- **Snack**: A slice of whole-grain toast with mashed avocado and lime.

- **Lunch**: Mediterranean chickpea salad with cucumbers, tomatoes, olives, and a tahini dressing.

- **Snack**: Fresh orange slices with a sprinkle of cinnamon.

- **Dinner**: Grilled shrimp with a wild rice and spinach pilaf.

- **Evening Drink**: Hibiscus tea.

Day 6

- **Breakfast**: Smoothie bowl with frozen mixed berries, almond milk, and granola topping.

- **Snack**: Sliced cucumbers and bell peppers with a yogurt dip.

- **Lunch**: Grilled salmon with a sweet potato and arugula salad.

- **Snack**: A boiled egg and a small handful of walnuts.

- **Dinner**: Turkey meatballs with spaghetti squash and a fresh tomato sauce.

- **Evening Drink**: Peppermint tea.

Day 7

- **Breakfast**: Buckwheat pancakes with a dollop of Greek yogurt and fresh blueberries.

- **Snack**: Sliced celery sticks with almond butter.

- **Lunch**: Miso soup with tofu, seaweed, and a side of steamed edamame.

- **Snack**: Fresh strawberries with a small handful of mixed nuts.

- **Dinner**: Grilled chicken skewers with a cucumber-tomato salad and quinoa.

- **Evening Drink**: Lemon balm tea.

Tips for Maximizing Energy and Revitalization

1. *Eat regularly:* Eat at the same times every day to keep your energy and blood sugar levels steady.
2. *Hydrate well:* Drink water every day and eat foods that are high in water.
3. *Eat protein at every meal.* This will give you long-lasting energy and help your cells heal.
4. *Stay away from things that drain your energy.* For example, eat less sugar, coffee, and processed foods that make you feel tired.

5. *Plan ahead:* Make meals ahead of time so you can always have healthy options during the week.

In Week 4, focus on meals that will help you feel better and give you more energy. This will help you finish the cellular health diet with renewed energy and the knowledge you need to live a healthier, more energized life.

Shopping List and Prep Tips for Success

To improve cell health through eating, make sure you have the right foods and know how to make them quickly. This section will assist you in identifying the items on your shopping list and provide tips to simplify the cooking process. Organizing your shopping list and making your meals ahead of time will save you time and make sure you always have healthy, energizing meals on hand.

Important Things to Put on Your Shopping List

We will build your weekly meal plans around the following items. They have many important nutrients, like antioxidants, beneficial fats, protein, fiber, and vitamins, which help keep cells healthy.

Proteins

- Fish and seafood, such as salmon, sardines, shrimp, and mackerel, are rich in omega-3 fatty acids.
- Poultry: Chicken breast and turkey
- Plant-based proteins: soybeans, chickpeas, lentils, black beans, quinoa, tofu, tempeh, and black beans
- Choose free-range or organic eggs.
- Some nuts and seeds that are beneficial for you are pumpkin seeds, flaxseeds, almonds, and walnuts.

Healthy Fats

- Avocados are a wonderful way to get fiber and healthy fats.
- Olive Oil: Use extra virgin olive oil for cooking or on top of food.

- Use coconut oil to cook or add it to drinks.
- Nuts and nut butters include peanut butter (without added sugar), walnuts, cashews, and almonds.
- Flaxseeds and chia seeds are excellent sources of omega-3 fatty acids.

Vegetables and Greens

- Leafy greens, like collard greens, kale, spinach, arugula, and Swiss chard
- Crispy vegetables: Brussels sprouts, broccoli, and cauliflower
- Root vegetables, like beets, sweet potatoes, and carrots
- Other vegetables include tomatoes, asparagus, bell peppers, cucumbers, and zucchini.

Fruits

- Berries: blackberries, raspberries, blueberries, and strawberries
- Citrus foods include oranges, lemons, and grapefruits.
- Avocados: They have a lot of beneficial fats.
- Bananas: A fantastic way to get potassium, which helps cells stay hydrated.

Whole Grains

- Quinoa is a gluten-free food that is high in protein.
- Brown rice is a beneficial way to get fiber.
- Oats: Prepare steel-cut oats for snacks or breakfast.
- Whole wheat: bread or pasta (if you can handle it).

Spices and Herbs

- Turmeric is a strong anti-inflammatory.
- Ginger helps the digestive system and lowers inflammation.
- Garlic: makes your defense system stronger
- Basil, parsley, and cilantro: fresh plants that add flavor and antioxidants

- Cayenne pepper, cinnamon, and cumin: for taste and to help the metabolism

Dairy or alternative foods to dairy

- Greek yogurt: For probiotics and calcium, opt for plain yogurt instead of sweetened ones.
- You can use unsweetened almond milk or other plant-based milks like coconut, cashew, or oat milk.
- Cheese: If desired, include a small amount of high-quality cheese such as feta or goat cheese.

Extras for the Pantry

- Apple cider vinegar helps the body get rid of toxins and digest food.
- If you want smooth stews and smoothies, use coconut milk.
- Nutritional yeast adds a cheesy taste and B vitamins to food.
- Use Himalayan pink salt and sea salt to maintain the balance of your electrolytes.
- Black pepper: helps the body absorb nutrients and adds flavor

Meal Prep Tips for Success

To stay on track with your cellular health diet, you need to plan and prepare your meals well. To make the process easier to handle and more fun, here are some tips.

Make a menu for the week.

Plan your meals for the week ahead of time. Knowing what you're going to cook ahead of time will save you time at the store and keep you from making incorrect choices during the week.

Use your meal plan as a guide: choose recipes and make a shopping list based on the week's food plan.

Batch cooking: To save time, make a lot of food at once for the week. For instance, make a big pot of quinoa, brown rice, or beans that you can use in different meals all week.

Get your shopping list in order

To save time while shopping, sort your ingredients into groups, like protein, veggies, grains, and herbs. You won't have to run around the store looking for different materials.

Eat whole foods: Choose fresh, whole foods that are beneficial for your cells.

Stay away from prepared foods. Prepared foods typically contain high levels of unhealthy fats, additives, and preservatives, all of which are detrimental to your cells.

Prepare the ingredients ahead of time.

Spend some time on your weekend (or day off) getting things ready so that cooking during the week is easier. You can do the following ahead of time:

Wash and cut up vegetables: Cut up carrots, onions, bell peppers, and leafy greens ahead of time. Keep them in sealed containers in the fridge so you can get to them quickly.

Cook vegetables and grains. Make a lot of quinoa, rice, lentils, and beans. If you want to make meals quickly, put them in the fridge or freezer.

Roast vegetables: For the week, roast a bunch of root veggies, like beets and sweet potatoes, that you can put in bowls or salads.

Get snacks ready. For quick snacks, divide up nuts and seeds into amounts or make energy bites with oats, nut butter, and chia seeds.

Get creative with leftovers

Make more of something so you can use the excess for another meal. As an example:

You can use any leftover roasted vegetables in salads, add them to a quinoa bowl, or have them for breakfast with eggs.

For a quick protein boost, add extra grilled chicken or fish to wraps, sandwiches, or salads.

Keep Your Kitchen Stocked with Essential Items

Ensure that your pantry is stocked with simple foods that you can use to prepare meals anywhere.

Cans of beans, such as chickpeas and black beans, are available

Canned tomato sauces and soups

You can eat seeds and nuts as a snack or add them to food.

Taste-enhancing spices like cinnamon, ginger, cumin, turmeric, and cumin

How to Save Time When Cooking

One-pot meals: There are meals that only need one pot, like soups, stews, and sauces. These take less time to make and clean up. You can make a lot of these meals at once and eat them over several days.

Use your slow cooker or Instant Pot. If you have one of these cooking tools, it can save you a lot of time when making soups, stews, and grains.

Smoothies: Put smoothie ingredients in bags ahead of time and freeze them. Just mix it with your favorite drink in the morning, and you have a quick and healthy meal or snack.

Following a cellular health diet will be easier and more fun if you plan your meals ahead of time, organize your shopping list, and prepare your ingredients ahead of time. With a little planning and the right ingredients, you can always make healthy, energizing meals that are beneficial for your cells and your general health.

PART 3:

LIFESTYLE ADJUSTMENTS TO ENHANCE CELLULAR HEALTH

CHAPTER 8

THE POWER OF MOVEMENT – EXERCISE FOR CELLULAR VITALITY

Movement is important for more than just looking and feeling fit. It feeds your cells and keeps them healthy. Working out has a big effect on the health and effectiveness of your cells, especially your mitochondria, which are like "powerhouses" because they make energy that keeps you alive. This chapter will talk about how exercise affects the health of cells, the kinds of workouts that help mitochondria work, and how to create a movement practice that makes you healthier and longer.

The Impact of Physical Activity on Cellular Health

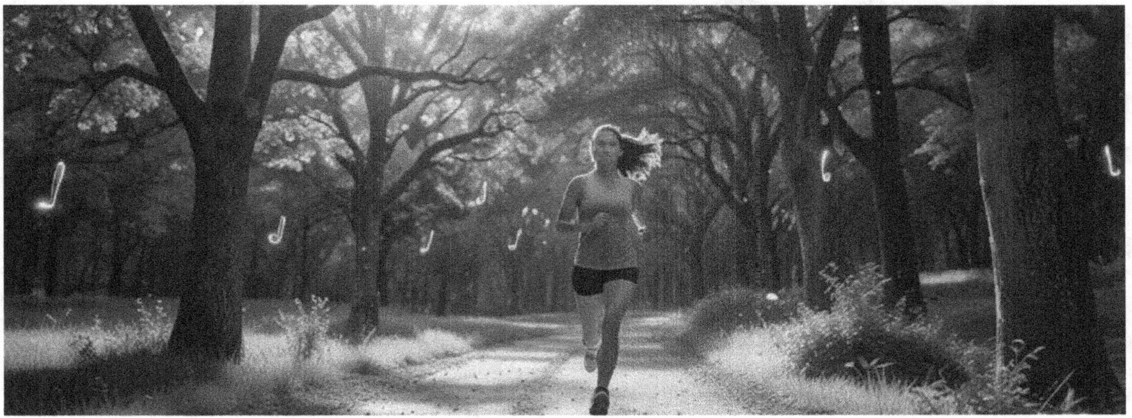

Physical exercise significantly impacts the level of cells, altering the way our bodies produce energy, repair damage, and maintain overall health. Exercise is beneficial for more than just your heart health and body tone; it also helps our cells, which are the building blocks of life.

Improved Mitochondrial Functioning

The mitochondria sometimes referred to as the "powerhouses" of the cell, produce adenosine triphosphate (ATP), the body's primary source of energy. Exercise speeds up a process known as mitochondrial biogenesis. This is the making of new mitochondria in cells.

The way it works: being active makes you need more energy. In response, cells adapt by producing more mitochondria, which enhances their ability to produce ATP. More mitochondria per cell mean more efficient energy production. This lets you be more active and last longer.

At the cellular level, mitochondrial biogenesis also slows down the aging process, since these parts of cells tend to break down with age and inaction. Regular exercise protects their function, which means they will keep making energy for life.

Less oxidative stress:

Exercise boosts the body's natural antioxidant protections, which fight free radicals. When cells breathe and other processes occur, they produce unstable chemicals known as free radicals. They can hurt DNA, proteins, and cells.

When you work out, your body uses more air, which makes more free radicals. However, regular exercise increases the production of antioxidant enzymes such as superoxide dismutase (SOD) and glutathione peroxidase.

Long-term benefit: This change makes the body better at fighting free radicals over time, which lowers oxidative stress and cell harm. This balance is important for keeping cells healthy and avoiding long-term illnesses.

Improved Cellular Waste Removal (Autophagy)

Autophagy is a process that cells use to get rid of broken parts, misfolded proteins, and harmful waste. Exercise helps this process happen.

Why it matters: Over time, cellular waste can build up and make cells less effective, which can lead to diseases like diabetes, cancer, and neurological disorders.

The role of exercise: Exercise starts autophagy in many organs, such as muscles, the liver, and the brain. This keeps cells "clean" and makes sure they work well.

By making autophagy better, exercise helps keep harmful substances from building up and encourages cell renewal, which makes the body healthier generally.

Enhanced Circulation and Nutrient Delivery

Being active makes the blood move faster, which means that oxygen and nutrients get to cells more quickly. This improved circulation directly enhances cellular performance.

Providing the body with the glucose and amino acids necessary for energy production and self-healing. More efficiently getting rid of waste like carbon dioxide and lactic acid.

Better circulation also raises the amount of oxygen in the tissues, which helps the mitochondria make energy and heals damaged cells.

Regulation of Inflammation

Chronic inflammation is a major cause of cell damage and the growth of many diseases, such as diabetes, heart disease, and cancer. Exercise causes changes in inflammatory markers, which naturally reduce inflammation in the body.

In the short term, intense exercise temporarily exacerbates inflammation as part of the healing process.

Long-term benefit: regular mild exercise lowers levels of inflammatory cytokines (like IL-6 and TNF-alpha) and raises levels of anti-inflammatory factors like interleukin-10.

This balance prevents long-term inflammation from damaging cells, improving the environment for cell function.

Protection against Cellular Aging

At the cellular level, physical exercise slows down aging by protecting the caps at the ends of chromosomes called telomeres.

What do telomeres do? Every time a cell splits, the telomeres get shorter. This makes cells age and stop working properly over time.

How exercise helps: Studies have shown that regular exercise can keep telomeres long by lowering toxic stress and speeding up the body's repair systems.

This effect slows down both the aging process and the chance of diseases that come with getting older.

Hormonal Balance and Cellular Function

Exercise alters the synthesis and regulation of hormones crucial for cell health.

Insulin sensitivity: Being active makes cells respond better to insulin, which makes it easier for cells to take in glucose and lowers the risk of getting diabetes.

Exercise raises brain-derived neurotrophic factor (BDNF) and other growth factors that help cells live and grow. This is especially true in the brain.

Being physically active on a regular basis has a huge impact on the health of cells. Exercise keeps cells in excellent shape by improving mitochondrial function, lowering oxidative stress, speeding up the removal of waste, and controlling inflammation. This means you'll have more energy, your immune system will be stronger, and your general health will be better. Whether you're walking, swimming, or lifting weights, each move you make makes your cells healthy and stronger.

Exercise That Supports Mitochondrial Function

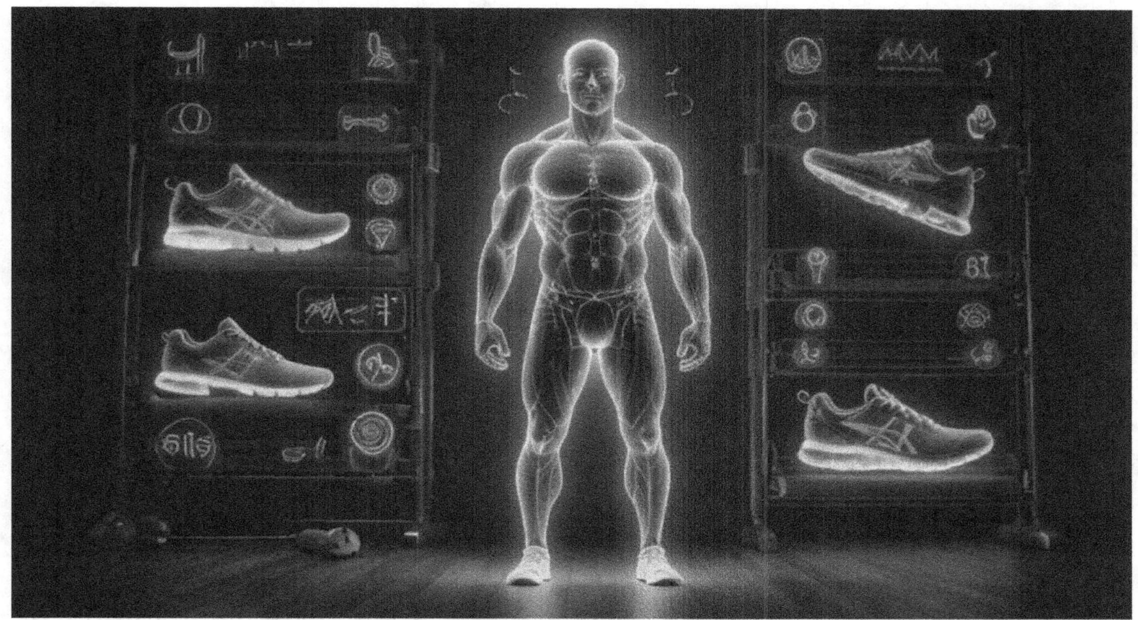

As the power plants that convert foods into adenosine triphosphate (ATP), the energy currency of cells, mitochondria play a crucial role in energy production. Exercise is one of the best ways to maintain mitochondrial function. Some types and levels of exercise can help mitochondria grow, fix, and work more efficiently, which improves the health of cells and their ability to make energy.

Aerobic Exercise: The Foundation for Mitochondrial Health

Aerobic exercise, often simply referred to as "cardio," is a crucial component of mitochondrial support because it directly tests the body's oxygen-dependent energy systems.

What happens: When you do physical exercise, your mitochondria have to make more ATP to meet your muscles' energy needs. This increased demand triggers the process of mitochondrial biogenesis, resulting in the creation of new mitochondria.

Some excellent examples of aerobic exercise are walking, jogging, swimming, cycling, and dancing.

Effort: For best results, work out at a moderate to vigorous level of effort, where you can still talk but feel your heart rate going up.

Long-term aerobic exercise raises both the number and quality of mitochondria, making them better at making energy and lowering the chance that they will stop working properly as you age.

High-Intensity Interval Training (HIIT): Turbocharging Mitochondrial Biogenesis

When you do high-intensity interval training (HIIT), you do short bursts of hard exercise followed by rest or low-intensity exercise.

Why it works: The intense effort of HIIT causes a short-term energy deficit that forces mitochondria to work at full capacity. This makes them grow and work better.

Benefits: Research has shown that HIIT can boost mitochondrial content and enzyme activity more than steady-state cardio.

Example of a HIIT workout:

To warm up, jog slowly for five minutes.

Interval: Run as fast as you can for 30 seconds.

Recovery: Take a 90-second walk or jog.

Repeat: every 6 to 8 minutes.

HIIT works especially well because it gives mitochondrial benefits in less time, which makes it perfect for people who are always on the go.

Resistance Training: Building Mitochondrial Strength

Strength training, which includes things like lifting weights, using resistance bands, and doing tasks with your own body, is also beneficial for mitochondrial health.

What it does: Resistance training increases the production of mitochondria in muscle cells, particularly in fast-twitch muscle fibers that aren't as active during aerobic exercise.

Key exercises: squats, deadlifts, push-ups, and rows with a support band work well.

How often should you work out? You should work out two to three times a week, focusing on big muscle groups.

When you do aerobic and interval training along with strength training, you get a well-rounded workout that helps mitochondria work properly in all muscle types.

Endurance Training: Sustained Energy for Mitochondria

Endurance exercise involves extended periods of moderately intense activity, which significantly enhance mitochondrial function and density.

How it works: Endurance exercise stresses the mitochondria over a longer period of time, which makes them more flexible and able to handle long-term energy needs.

Long-distance jogging, cycling, or rowing for 45 to 60 minutes are all examples.

Adaptation: Over time, physical training raises the amount of mitochondria in muscles, which makes them stronger and less tired.

Functional and Dynamic Exercises

Even though yoga, Pilates, and tai chi may not look as intense as other types of exercise, they can still help keep your mitochondria healthy.

How they help: These actions improve oxygen delivery, blood flow, and nutrient uptake by cells, all of which make mitochondria work better.

As an added bonus, they reduce stress, which is known to negatively impact mitochondrial function by elevating oxidative stress levels.

Incorporating functional and dynamic movements into your practice can help both high-intensity and endurance training in different ways.

Exercise and Mitochondrial Repair

Regular exercise not only accelerates the production of new mitochondria but also aids in the repair of damaged mitochondria. Mitophagy, a process, recycles mitochondria that aren't functioning properly.

How it starts: Both aerobic and resistance workouts start processes that help mitophagy happen. This keeps cells' mitochondria healthy and working.

Exercise gets rid of harmed mitochondria and stops the buildup of cell debris that could slow down energy production and lead to diseases that come with getting older.

Tips for Optimizing Exercise for Mitochondrial Health

To get the most out of exercise's effects on mitochondrial function, keep these things in mind:

Consistency is key: you need to work out at least four to five days a week to get long-lasting mitochondrial effects.

Mix it up: Do a range of workouts, such as aerobics, HIIT, and strength training, to work on different parts of mitochondrial function.

Drink plenty of water. For mitochondria to make ATP properly, they need water. Before, during, and after activity, make sure you drink plenty of water.

Help the body recover: getting enough rest and sleep helps the body heal and adjust, which is beneficial for mitochondrial health.

One of the best ways to improve mitochondrial function, boost energy production, and keep cells healthy in general is to exercise. By doing a mix of aerobic, high-intensity, and strength training, you can improve the efficiency, growth, and repair of your mitochondria. Over time, these habits help your cells stay healthy and strong, which supports your vitality and life.

Cardiovascular, Strength, and Flexibility Routines for Optimal Cellular Energy

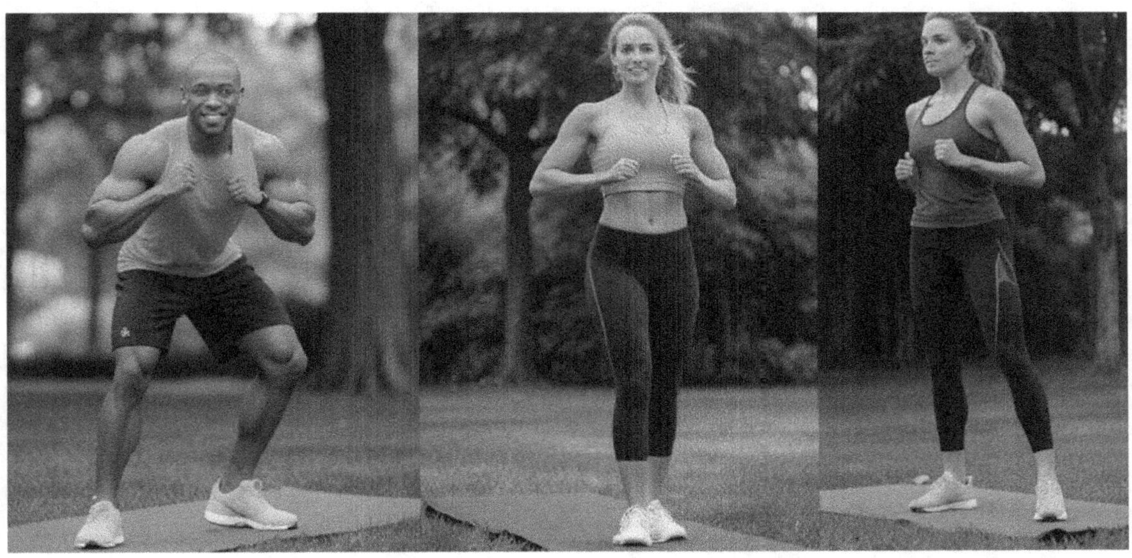

Including cardiovascular training, strength-building activities, and flexibility exercises in a well-rounded exercise routine can enhance cell energy production and improve overall health. Each type of exercise is beneficial for the body in its own way, and they all work together to improve circulation, keep cells healthy, and make mitochondria work better.

Cardiovascular Exercise: Energizing the Mitochondria

Cardiovascular exercise is essential for keeping the heart healthy, improving circulation, and getting more oxygen to cells. All these elements are essential for the proper functioning of mitochondria and the production of ATP.

Benefits of Cellular Power

- It increases the density and efficiency of the mitochondria in muscle cells.
- Makes it easier for cells to take in and move oxygen, which is needed for aerobic energy creation.
- Lowers reactive stress, which helps cells heal and last longer.

Different kinds of Cardiovascular Exercise

- *Walking is an easy-to-do*, low-impact exercise that improves circulation and builds muscle over time.
- *Running or jogging:* These are higher-intensity exercises that test your heart and lungs and boost mitochondrial biogenesis.
- *Swimming* is a fantastic way to work out your whole body and get more air while being gentle on your joints.
- *Riding:* Especially in interval-based routines, riding makes lower body muscles stronger and boosts cardiovascular output.
- *Dancing:* This activity combines cardio with fun and imagination, and it helps you burn calories over a long period of time.

Example of a Routine

- Three to five days a week.
- Level of intensity: moderate (heart rate up, but you can still talk) or intense (sweating, out of breath).
- Time: 20 to 60 minutes, based on how fit you are.

Strength Training: Building Power at the Cellular Level

The main goals of strength training, also called resistance training, are to build muscle mass, make bones stronger, and improve the function of mitochondria in muscle fibers. Strength training targets fast-twitch muscle fibers, which are less active during aerobic activity, allowing it to complement cardiovascular exercise.

Benefits for Cellular Energy

- It facilitates the growth of mitochondria in muscle cells.
- It enhances the function of insulin, enabling the body to utilize glucose for energy more effectively.
- Lowers the buildup of fat, which can make cells less effective.

Types of Strength Exercises

- *Exercises you can do with your own body:* pushups, push-ups, squats, and lunges.
- *Weightlifting:* working out certain muscle groups with dumbbells, barbells, or resistance tools.
- *Resistance* bands are lightweight and effective for total body workouts.
- *When you do jump-based workouts*, like box jumps, you build muscle power and make your mitochondria work better.

Routine Example

- Twice or three times a week
- For building muscle, do 8–12 reps, and for stamina, do 15–20 reps.
- Sets: two to four per practice.
- Rest for one to two minutes in between sets.

Flexibility and Mobility Training: Supporting Cellular Flow

Mobility and flexibility exercises increase the body's range of motion, lower the chance of injury, and help tissues get the blood they need. These movements, in conjunction with cardio and strength training, facilitate the production of energy in cells by ensuring proper delivery of oxygen and nutrients.

Benefits for Cellular Energy

- Improves blood flow and the release of nutrients to cells.

- Lowers worry and tension, which can make mitochondrial function worse.
- Maintaining healthy joints enables you to move more effectively during other workouts.

Types of Flexibility and Mobility Exercises

- *Yoga:* This form of exercise combines stretching with awareness to help reduce stress and improve circulation.
- *Dynamic stretching* involves movements such as arm circles and leg swings that prepare muscles for exercise.
- *Static Stretching:* Hold stretches for 20 to 30 seconds after a workout to make muscles more flexible.
- *Foam rolling:* It loosens up tight muscles, which helps circulation and healing.
- If you do *Pilates or Tai Chi,* focus on slow, simple moves that make you more flexible and strengthen your core.

Routine Example

- How often: Every day or right after each workout.
- Each practice lasts 10 to 20 minutes.

Combining the Three Components for Cellular Vitality

A complete exercise plan includes power, cardio, and flexibility exercises to improve health and cell energy.

Weekly Plan

Day	Activity
Monday	30 minutes of brisk walking or light jogging (cardio) + 10 minutes of yoga (flexibility).
Tuesday	Resistance training: squats, push-ups, and resistance band rows (strength).

Wednesday	40 minutes of cycling or swimming (cardio).
Thursday	Yoga or Pilates session (flexibility) + foam rolling.
Friday	25 minutes of HIIT (cardio) + planks and lunges (strength).
Saturday	Endurance cardio: 60-minute hike or long-distance cycling.
Sunday	Rest day with light stretching or tai chi (flexibility).

Tips to Get Long-Lasting Cellular Benefits

- Find a satisfactory balance between intensity and recovery. Cells can get damaged from overtraining. Include days off and things that aren't too hard.
- Be Consistent: Doing things regularly is better for you than doing short, rigorous workouts here and there.
- Feed Your Body: A nutrient-dense diet and regular exercise will give your cells the fuel they need to grow and fix themselves.
- Pay Attention to Your Body: Change how hard you work out and how long you do it based on your energy level and physical health.

The Benefits of Cellular Health

Including strength, cardio, and flexibility exercises in your daily routine improves the health of your mitochondria, boosts cellular energy production, and increases your general vitality. By doing these activities together, you not only improve the function of your cells, but you also improve your endurance, strength, and movement, which will help you live a longer, healthier life.

How to Start and Maintain a Movement Practice

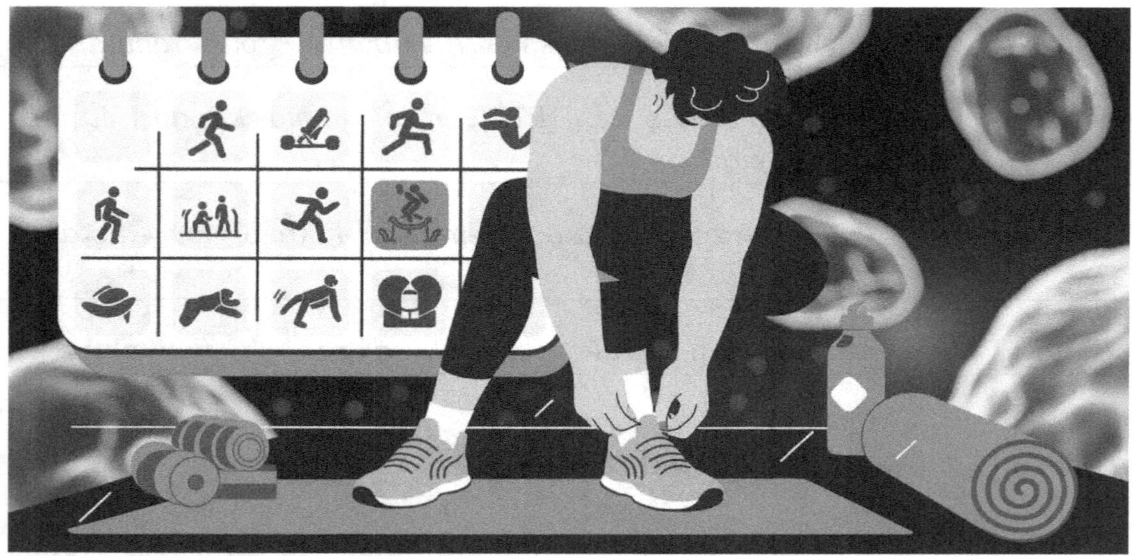

Starting and sticking with a movement routine is important for maintaining healthy cells and general vitality over time. To get benefits like better mitochondrial function, more cellular energy, and less oxidative stress, consistency is more important than effort. This guide gives you steps you can take right now to make exercise a part of your daily life and keep it up for good.

Starting Your Movement Practice

Set Realistic Goals

Determine your "why": identify what motivates you, such as increased energy, improved health, or a higher quality of life.

Start small. Set goals that you can reach, like walking for 10 minutes every day or doing a short yoga exercise.

Tell me more: Set SMART goals, which stand for Specific, Measurable, Achievable, Relevant, and Time-bound." It could be, "I will jog for 20 minutes, three times a week.

Pick Things You Like To Do.

Sustainability is guaranteed by personal choice. Choose things to do that make you feel good, like Pilates, dancing, swimming, or hikes.

Try new things: Do a variety of things to find what you enjoy.

Set Up a Routine.

Make exercise a regular part of your life. Plan to move around at certain times of the day.

Start with low-frequency lessons, such as twice or three times a week, and gradually increase the frequency to more frequent ones.

Get your Environment Ready.

Pick a place to work out, even if it's just a small room at home.

Buy clothes that are simple to wear and shoes that support your feet, as well as basic exercise gear like yoga mats and resistance bands.

Learn the Proper Technique

Seek guidance from a professional or an online lesson to ensure proper form and reduce your risk of injury.

Begin with beginner-friendly classes or sessions tailored to your fitness level.

Overcoming Common Barriers

Not Enough Time

Add some movement to your day. For example, park farther away, take the stairs, or do 5-minute workout bursts.

Focus on getting the most out of your workouts. High-intensity interval training (HIIT) and compound strength exercises get you the most out of your time.

No Motivation

Work out with a friend or sign up for a class to keep yourself accountable and inspired.

Reward yourself: As a reward for being consistent, give yourself small things like a bath or a new exercise accessory.

Physical Limitations

Change the exercises to fit your level of fitness. You can do low-impact exercises like chair yoga, aqua aerobics, or walks.

If necessary, consult a healthcare professional about creating a personalized plan.

Keeping up with your Movement Practice

Mix Things Up.

Switch between strength, cardio, and flexibility workouts to avoid getting bored and work out a variety of muscle groups.

Do things that fit the season, like skiing in the winter, hiking in the summer, or working out inside when it rains.

Keep Track Of Your Progress.

Keep track of your activity levels, progress, and goals with fitness apps or journals.

Celebrate your wins: Reward yourself when you reach your goals, like running your first mile or working out every day for a week.

Adapt to the Changes in your Life.

Stay flexible: Change your schedule to fit work, family, or trip plans.

Make a plan for what you will do if you are unable to attend a scheduled workout. If you miss one, do a quick 10-minute exercise instead.

Keep Going.

Give yourself new goals. For example, join a charity run, learn a new sport, or try to get better at advanced yoga poses.

Find motivation by reading books, listening to podcasts, or following fitness celebrities who inspire you.

Practical Tips for Long-Term Success

Make It Convenient

Pick places that are easy to get to, like a home gym or a park close by.

Make plans ahead of time. Lay out your workout clothes the night before or prepare your gym bag for the day after work.

Incorporate Movement Into Daily Life

Do more than one thing at once. For example, do squats while watching TV or stretching while the water boils.

During breaks at work, take short walks or do workouts at your desk.

Be Consistent

Work on making it a habit: try to do it regularly, even if the lessons are short.

Use triggers: Connect your workouts to things you do every day, like going for a walk after breakfast or stretching before bed.

The Cellular Health Benefits of a Sustained Movement Practice

Enhanced Cellular Energy

Regular exercise encourages mitochondrial biogenesis, which over time raises the production of energy in cells.

Improved Longevity

Working out lowers oxidative stress and inflammation, two things that make cells age faster.

Stronger Resilience

Regular exercise teaches your body to deal with stress, heal faster, and keep working at its best.

Example Beginner Movement Schedule

Day	Activity	Duration
Monday	10-minute brisk walk + 5 minutes of stretching	15 minutes
Tuesday	Bodyweight exercises (squats, push-ups, planks)	15 minutes
Wednesday	Gentle yoga or Pilates session	20 minutes
Thursday	Rest day with light stretching	10 minutes
Friday	HIIT session (e.g., 30 seconds on, 30 seconds rest)	15 minutes
Saturday	Long walk or swim	30 minutes
Sunday	Active recovery: foam rolling or tai chi	20 minutes

Getting into and sticking with a movement practice is a process that changes over time. You can unlock the deep cellular benefits of regular physical exercise by making goals that are attainable, finding activities that you enjoy, and sticking to them. Don't forget that it's not about being great, but about getting better. Even small, regular efforts can improve the health and vigor of cells and the body as a whole.

CHAPTER 9

SLEEP AND CELLULAR HEALTH – THE UNDERRATED VITALITY BOOST

Not everyone thinks of sleep as important, but it's one of the best ways to improve cell health and vitality. While you sleep, your body does important things like repair, regeneration, and cleansing that set the stage for optimal health. This chapter goes into detail about the complex connection between sleep and cellular health, highlighting its huge effect and giving useful advice for getting the most out of restful sleep.

How Sleep Affects Cellular Repair and Regeneration

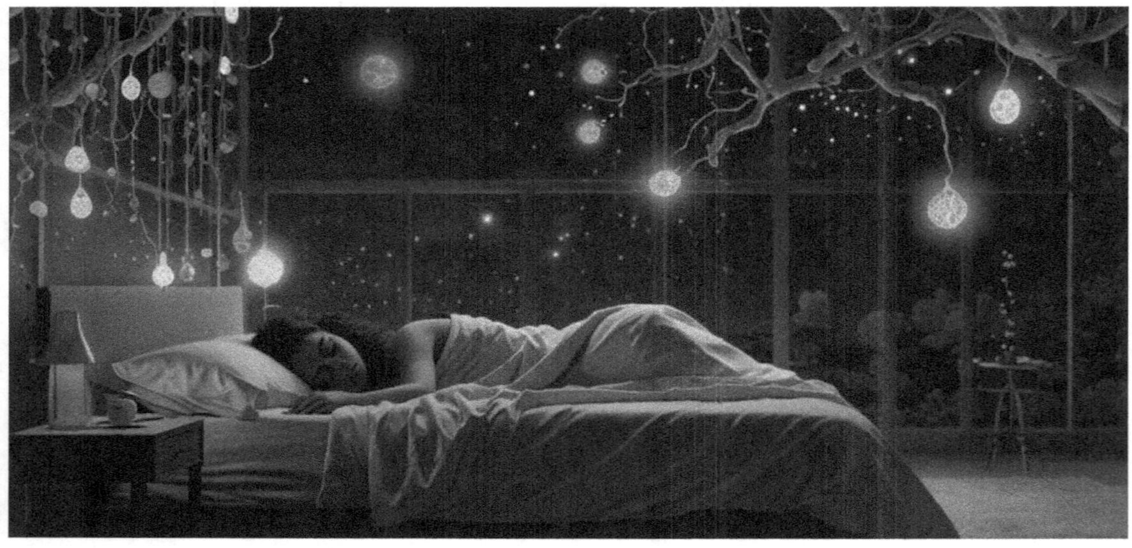

Getting enough sleep is essential for keeping cells healthy because it helps the body mend, regenerate, and rejuvenate itself. While you sleep, your body goes into a state of restorative activity, focusing on tasks that keep cells healthy and your general health in excellent shape. Let's look into these processes in more detail:

Tissue Regeneration and Healing

Sleep is important for healing and growth because it helps muscles heal and grow again.

Release of Growth Hormone: The pituitary gland releases growth hormone while you are in deep sleep. This hormone helps the body make more proteins. This is crucial for repairing damaged muscle fibers, tissues, and cells.

Healing Wounds: Adequate sleep accelerates the healing process of wounds. Studies have shown that getting enough sleep helps people heal from accidents faster by speeding up the production of collagen and cells.

DNA Repair

Every day, toxins in the surroundings, UV light, and metabolic processes hurt the DNA in every cell. During sleep, you can fix these mistakes:

Reversal of DNA Damage: While you sleep, special cell processes find and fix DNA strand breaks and oxidative damage. This stops changes that can cause long-term illnesses like cancer.

Genomic Stability: Getting enough sleep keeps your DNA stable, which is important for cells to work properly and for you to live a long time.

Immune System Optimization

Sleep makes it easier for the immune system to fight off germs and fix damage to cells caused by stress.

Cytokines are proteins that regulate the immune system's response. Their production goes up while you sleep, which helps the immune system find and kill dangerous invaders and heal damaged tissues.

White Blood Cell Activity: White blood cells, especially T-cells and natural killer cells, become more active while you sleep. These cells are crucial for finding and killing damaged or sick cells.

Detoxification and Waste Removal

The body speeds up its cleansing processes while you sleep to get rid of waste from cells.

Detox for the brain: While you sleep, your brain's glymphatic system works very hard. It eliminates waste products such as beta-amyloid plaques, associated with neurological diseases such as Alzheimer's.

Cellular Autophagy: Autophagy is a process that cells use to recycle and get rid of broken parts, making room for new cells to grow. This is especially helpful for keeping chronic diseases at bay and slowing down the aging process.

Energy Recovery and Mitochondrial Function

You need to sleep in order for your cells' energy producers to function again.

Maintenance of the mitochondria: During sleep, the mitochondria repair themselves to enhance their energy production during the day. This lowers oxidative stress and helps cells work better generally.

ATP Replenishment: During sleep, cells replenish ATP, their energy currency. This lets cells work at their best when they wake up.

Hormonal Balance

Hormones directly affect how cells heal and grow back, and sleep is necessary to keep them in balance.

Lowering cortisol: Sleep lowers cortisol levels, which is a stress hormone that can stop cells from healing if it stays high for a long time.

Making melanin: This sleep hormone controls the sleep-wake cycle and is also a strong antioxidant that helps DNA repair and protects cells from environmental damage.

Reduction of Inflammation

Chronic inflammation accelerates the aging and damage of cells. Inflammation can be reduced by sleep by:

Cytokine Regulation: When you sleep, your body makes less of the cytokines that cause inflammation and more of the ones that stop it. This keeps your immune system in balance.

Lessening of oxidative stress: Sleep lowers oxidative damage, a major cause of inflammation, by protecting mitochondria from damage and getting rid of free radicals.

Cognitive and Emotional Repair

Sleep facilitates the repair of brain cells, promoting both mental and emotional well-being.

Neuron Restoration: While you sleep, neural cells fix themselves, which makes it easier to remember things, learn new things, and use your brain in general.

Controlling your emotions: Sleep resets the balance of neurotransmitters like dopamine and serotonin, which are important for keeping your emotions stable and strong.

Enhanced Telomere Maintenance

Telomeres are caps that guard the ends of chromosomes. Stress and aging cause cells to shorten. Getting enough sleep helps them stay long.

Slow Telomere Shortening: Regular sleep slows down the rate of telomere shortening, which is associated with longer lifespans and a lower risk of chronic diseases.

The complicated link between sleep and cell recovery shows how important it is for health and well-being. By making getting enough sleep a priority, you give your body the chance to do important maintenance tasks that keep your cells healthy, strong, and ready to support your vitality and life.

The Role of Deep Sleep in Longevity and Resilience

Some people also call this stage of sleep "slow-wave sleep" (SWS). It is the most restful. During this time, your brain and body are doing important things that help keep your cells healthy, your hormones in balance, and your general strength, all of which are important for living a long life. Let's look at how getting deep sleep can help you live longer and healthier.

Cellular Repair and Regeneration

The body repairs and replaces cells damaged by daily activities and environmental stress during deep sleep.

Protein Synthesis: Growth hormone, which increases during deep sleep, speeds up protein synthesis. This helps heal tissues, recover muscles, and renew skin, which are all important for slowing down the aging process.

Cellular processes during deep sleep can repair damage to DNA. This prevents genetic mutations that could cause chronic diseases or faster aging.

Hormonal Regulation

During deep sleep, the balance of key chemicals makes you stronger and helps you live longer.

Release of the Growth Hormone: Growth hormone is one of the most important hormones for repair, and it is highest during deep sleep. This helps cells grow back and the body stay healthy overall.

Cortisol Suppression: Deep sleep lowers cortisol levels. Cortisol is a stress hormone that speeds up aging and makes inflammation worse when it stays high for a long time.

Melatonin is a powerful antioxidant that combats free radicals and protects cells from environmental damage during sleep.

Brain Detoxification and Cognitive Longevity

Deep sleep is an important part of keeping your brain healthy, which is important for staying strong and living a long life.

Activity of the Glymphatic System: This system primarily eliminates waste, such as beta-amyloid clumps, during deep sleep. These plaques are associated with neurodegenerative illnesses like Alzheimer's.

Neuronal Maintenance: As you age, deep sleep facilitates the repair and pruning of neural links, thereby maintaining your memory and cognitive function.

Immune System Optimization

Deep sleep makes the immune system stronger, which helps fight off infections and long-term illnesses.

Production of Cytokines: Deep sleep produces anti-inflammatory cytokines that reduce systemic inflammation, which accelerates aging and increases the risk of illness.

Activation of T-Cells: Sleep increases the activity of T-cells, which are essential for identifying and eliminating abnormal or sick cells.

Metabolic and Mitochondrial Health

Deep sleep is an important part of keeping metabolic and energy-producing processes running smoothly, which affects the health of cells.

Insulin Sensitivity: Getting a lot of deep sleep makes insulin work better, which lowers the chance of metabolic diseases like type 2 diabetes.

Mitochondrial Function: Mitochondria fix and rejuvenate themselves during deep sleep, making sure that the body makes the most energy possible and lowering oxidative stress.

Keeping Telomeres Healthy

Ageing closely correlates with the caps that protect chromosomes, known as telomeres. They stay healthy because deep sleep helps them.

Maintenance of Telomere Length: Research indicates that individuals who get enough deep sleep typically have longer telomeres, which are associated with slower cell aging and longer life spans.

Managing stress and maintaining emotional stability

Deep sleep makes you emotionally stronger, which has a direct effect on your health and how fast you age.

Recovery from stress: deep sleep helps the brain deal with and heal from mental stress, which lowers the body's long-term effects.

Mood Regulation: Deep sleep helps keep your emotions stable by recovering neurotransmitter levels like serotonin and dopamine. This is beneficial for your mental and physical health.

Enhanced Cardiovascular Health

Getting enough deep sleep is important for heart health, which in turn affects how long you live.

Controlling blood pressure: Low blood pressure and heart rate happen during deep sleep, giving the heart and blood vessels a much-needed break.

Controlling cholesterol: Deep sleep helps control lipids, which means that harmful cholesterol doesn't build up as much and can cause heart disease.

Reduction of Chronic Inflammation

Chronic inflammation is a big cause of aging and illness, and getting enough deep sleep can help reduce it.

Lowers C-reactive protein levels: Getting enough deep sleep lowers C-reactive protein levels, a sign of inflammation associated with heart disease and other age-related issues.

Better anti-inflammatory processes: When you're in a deep sleep, your body makes more anti-inflammatory molecules, which helps keep your internal environment better and less inflammatory.

Improved Longevity via Sleep Consistency

Getting into deep sleep on a regular basis is beneficial for your health and your hormonal rhythm.

Circadian Rhythm Synchronization: Deep sleep synchronizes with the body's circadian rhythm, ensuring correct hormone release and optimal cell function to promote a longer lifespan.

Long-Term Benefits: Regular deep sleep builds tolerance over time, which lowers the risk of chronic diseases and helps people live longer.

Useful Tips to Enhance Sleep

To maximize the life-enhancing benefits of deep sleep, consider the following actions:

Stick to a regular sleep schedule. This means going to bed and getting up at the same time every day.

Create the Best Environment for Sleep: To get a relaxing night's sleep, keep your room cool, dark, and quiet.

Limit stimulants: Don't eat or drink a lot of caffeine, nicotine, or heavy foods right before bed.

Use relaxation techniques. Doing yoga or meditation before bed can help calm your mind and get your body ready for a deep sleep.

Deep sleep is more than just a place to rest at night; it is a crucial time for fixing cells, cleaning out the brain, and keeping hormones in check. By making deep sleep a priority, you invest in your body's longevity and strength, setting the stage for a better, more fulfilling life.

Tips for Improving Sleep Quality and Restorative Rest

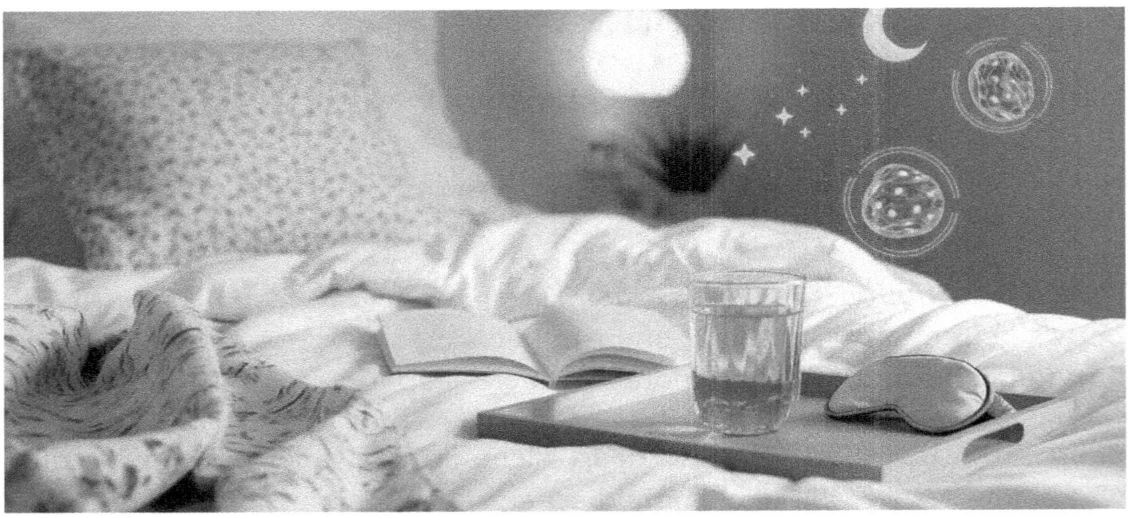

Cellular health relies heavily on good sleep for repair, regeneration, and overall health. If you don't get enough adequate sleep, these processes can't work as well, leaving your body open to tiredness, sickness, and aging faster. Here are numerous tips to improve your sleep quality and achieve truly restful sleep.

Make a Regular Schedule For Sleeping.

The body's internal clock, or circadian rhythm, is in sync when you sleep at regular times. This helps you get deep, restful sleep.

Go to bed and wake up at the same time every day. Being consistent lets your body know when to release hormones like melatonin that help you sleep.

Stick to the same schedule on the weekends. Don't stay up too late or sleep too late, as this can mess up your circadian cycle.

Create a Sleep-Conducive Environment

The right place to sleep can make a huge difference in how well you sleep.

Keep your bedroom dark. To do this, use blackout curtains or an eye mask to block out light. This is because darkness triggers your body to produce more melatonin.

Keep the room cool. The best setting for sleep is usually between 60°F and 67°F (15°C and 19°C). A cool room helps the body's temperature drop naturally while you sleep.

Lessen the noise: To block out annoying sounds, use earplugs or a white noise machine.

Buy comfortable bedding. Pick a mattress that supports you, sheets that let air flow, and pillows that are right for the way you sleep.

Control the Amount of Light

Light exposure is a vital part of controlling your sleep-wake cycle.

Get Natural Light During the Day: Sunlight, especially early in the morning, makes your circadian cycle stronger.

Limit blue light at night. Screens like phones, computers, and TVs give off blue light, which stops melatonin from working. Put on glasses that block blue light or turn on "night mode" on your gadgets.

Improve your Evening Habits

The things you do in the hours before bed have a big effect on how easily you can fall asleep.

Set up a wind-down routine. Doing relaxing things like reading, breathing, or taking a warm bath will tell your body it's time to sleep.

Don't do activities that will stimulate you. For example, don't do intense exercise or have talks that will make you feel awful right before bed.

Don't use too much nicotine or caffeine. These are both triggers that can make it difficult to sleep, so stay away from them in the afternoon and evening.

Don't drink alcohol before bed. Alcohol may help you fall asleep at first, but it wakes you up during deep sleep and REM sleep.

Give your Body What It Needs To Sleep.

What you eat and when you eat can affect how well you sleep.

Don't eat big meals right before bed. This can cause discomfort and hinder your ability to fall asleep.

Eat foods that help you sleep. Turkey, almonds, cherries, and bananas are all high in tryptophan, magnesium, and melatonin, which are all chemicals that help you relax.

Stay hydrated: Drink water all day, but cut back on how much you drink before bed to avoid waking up in the middle of the night.

Use Techniques for Relaxation.

Anxiety and stress make it difficult to sleep. It can make a big difference to learn techniques that calm the mind.

Do mindfulness meditation. Body scan exercises and focusing on your breath can help you relax and prepare for sleep.

Try progressive muscle relaxation. Tensing and resting each muscle group one at a time can help you relax and release stress.

Try aromatherapy. Smells like lavender and chamomile can help you feel calm and sleep better.

Align with Your Circadian Rhythm

Working with your body's natural rhythms can help you sleep better and have more energy.

Sleep in Line with Your Chronotype: If you naturally sleep late or early, try to plan your sleep around those times as much as possible.

Optimize your sleep cycles by aiming for complete 90-minute sleep cycles. You feel better when you wake up at the end of a cycle instead of in the middle.

Deal with the causes of Sleep Disorders

If you make changes to your lifestyle but still can't get adequate sleep, you might have a sleep problem.

Talk to a medical professional: If you have sleep apnea, restless leg syndrome, or sleeplessness, you may need medical help.

Think about cognitive behavioral treatment for insomnia (CBT-I). This type of treatment helps people who have trouble sleeping change the negative thoughts and actions that are keeping them up at night.

Limit Naps During the Day.

Short naps can help you feel better, but taking too many or too late in the day can make it difficult to sleep at night.

*Take short naps—ten to twenty minutes is ideal—*so you don't fall into deep sleep, which can make you feel sleepy.

Nap Early in the Day: If you want to be able to fall asleep at night without any problems, don't nap after 3 p.m.

Use Supplements Wisely

While supplements can aid in sleep, you shouldn't use them in place of healthy sleep habits.

Melatonin helps keep the sleep-wake cycle in balance, which is helpful for people who have jet lag or work shifts.

Magnesium: It aids in relaxation by maintaining the proper function of your muscles and calming your nervous system.

Valerian Root and Chamomile: These are natural herbs that can help you relax a little.

Monitor and Modify your Sleeping Habits.

Check in and improve your sleeping habits on a regular basis to get the most out of refreshing sleep.

Use sleep tracking tools. Apps or devices can monitor your sleep quality and highlight areas for improvement.

Make changes based on events in your life: If you're under a lot of stress, going on a trip, or your schedule changes, you may need to temporarily alter how you sleep.

Do Regular Physical Activities.

Getting some exercise is one of the best things you can do to improve your sleep.

Work out early: Working out in the morning or afternoon helps you sleep better at night.

Do some relaxing things in the evening. For example, gentle yoga or stretching can help you relax and let go of stress.

To get better sleep, you need to pay attention to your surroundings, your habits, your diet, and your attitude. By using these tips, you can make a sleep schedule that not only helps you sleep better at night but also improves the health of your cells, giving you more energy, making you stronger, and making you live longer. Putting restorative sleep first is an important thing you can do for your physical, social, and emotional health.

CHAPTER 10

STRESS MANAGEMENT – PROTECTING YOUR CELLS FROM OVERLOAD

Today's life is full of things that can be stressful, like difficult work and personal duties. Stress is a normal reaction to problems, but too much of it can damage the health of cells. This chapter discusses the impact of stress on cells, provides practical stress management techniques, and explores how to apply these techniques in daily life to maintain cell health.

The Effects of Chronic Stress on Cellular Health

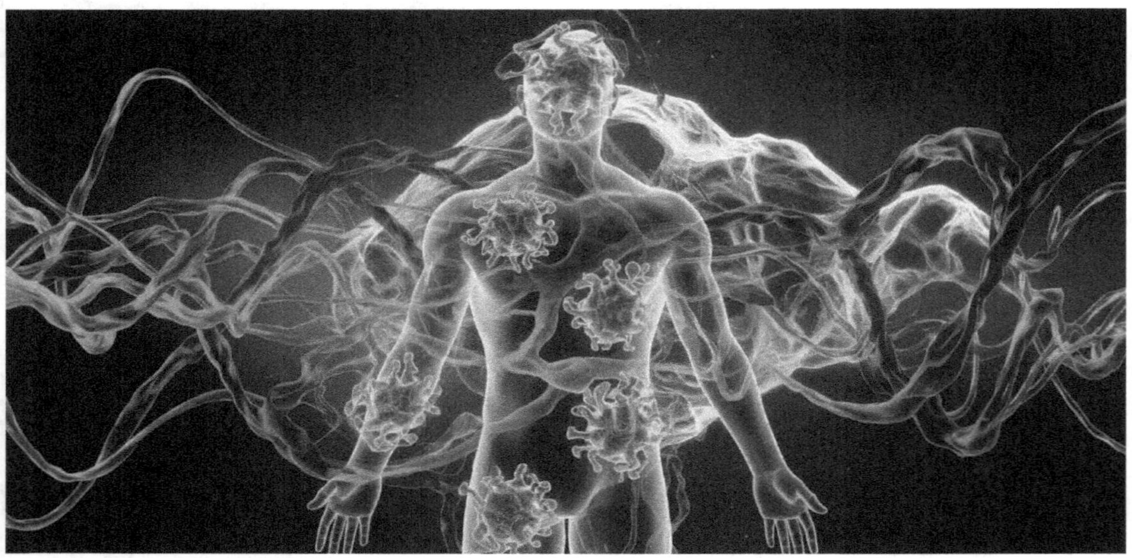

Stress is a normal reaction to the problems we face in life, but when it lasts for a long time, it hurts our cells in deep and important ways. Long-term worry sets off a chain of physiological responses that can hurt cells, make it harder for them to work, and speed up the aging and disease processes. Understand these effects to realize how important stress management is.

Elevated Cortisol and Cellular Damage

- Adrenal cells sometimes referred to as the "stress hormone," release cortisol when we experience high levels of stress. While cortisol levels that stay high for a long time can help with short-term worry, they hurt cells in the long term:
- *Shortening of telomeres:* Telomeres are caps that protect the ends of chromosomes and keep genetic information safe. Stress that lasts for a long time speeds up telomere shortening, which is a sign of aging cells. If your telomeres are shorter as you age, you are more likely to develop heart disease, diabetes, and cancer.
- *DNA Damage:* High amounts of cortisol make DNA strand breaks more likely, which makes it harder for cells to copy themselves and fix themselves. This could cause changes and sickness.
- *Reduced cell growth:* Stress inhibits the production of growth factors such as brain-derived neurotrophic factor (BDNF), essential for cells to repair and regenerate.

Increased Oxidative Stress

Reactive oxygen species (ROS) and the body's antioxidants, which can neutralize them, are mismatched. This leads to oxidative stress. Long-term stress increases ROS generation by:

- *Inflammation:* Stress sets off paths that cause inflammation and releases molecules that make ROS.
- *Mitochondrial Dysfunction:* When cells are under stress, the energy-making mitochondria get too busy and release too many ROS.

Cellular Consequences:

- Lipid peroxidation hurts cell walls, which makes cells less stable.
- Protein oxidation changes enzymes and structural proteins, which makes it harder for cells to work.
- Damage to DNA makes it harder for cells to divide and fix themselves, which could cause changes.

Impaired Immune System Function

Stress changes the immune system in ways that have a direct effect on the health of cells:

Suppressed Immune Cells: Long-term cortisol makes white blood cells less active, which makes it harder for the body to fight infections and fix damaged tissues.

Increased inflammatory cytokines: Stress increases the release of pro-inflammatory cytokines, which, if unchecked, can harm healthy cells and tissues.

These effects lower the defenses of cells, making them more likely to get sick from pathogens and environmental chemicals.

Disrupted Mitochondrial Function

Mitochondria are what give cells their energy. Long-term stress affects their ability to do things by:

- *Less ATP Production:* Stress reduces the effectiveness of oxidative phosphorylation, the process by which mitochondria produce ATP, the energy source for cells.
- *Damage to the mitochondria:* Stress-induced ROS damage mitochondrial membranes and DNA, causing the body to use less energy and increasing the likelihood of metabolic diseases and fatigue.

Cellular Aging and Senescence

Stress accelerates the aging process.

- Changes in epigenetics: Prolonged anxiety alters the epigenome, a collection of chemical alterations on DNA that regulate gene expression. These changes can turn off genes that help with repair and on genes that make inflammation worse.
- Cellular Senescence: Cells can enter senescence, a state where they can't grow or work properly, when they are under a lot of

stress for a long time. Senescent cells release inflammatory molecules that can damage tissues and lead to age-related diseases.

Effects on Brain Cells: Brain Science

Neurons are especially affected by stress, which can lead to

- *Less Neurogenesis:* Stress stops the growth of new neurons, especially in the hippocampus, a part of the brain that helps with learning and remembering.
- *Increased neuroinflammation:* Stress-induced inflammation damages neurons and disrupts brain networks.
- *Cognitive Decline:* These effects make it harder to remember things, concentrate, and control your emotions over time.

Altered Cellular Communication

Stress changes the way cells talk to each other, which makes it harder for them to work together to fix tissues and fight off infections.

Some important delays are:

- *Hormonal Imbalances:* Stress changes the way hormones talk to each other, which can affect insulin sensitivity and thyroid function, both of which are important for cell metabolism.
- *Ineffective autophagy:* Autophagy is the mechanism through which cells eliminate damaged components. When cells experience high levels of stress, their autophagy function is compromised, leading to the accumulation of waste products and toxins.

Increased Risk of Chronic Diseases

Over time, the impact of stress on cells increases the risk of developing long-term illnesses.

- *Heart and blood vessel diseases:* inflammation and oxidative damage caused by stress make angina and high blood pressure more likely.
- *Metabolic Disorders:* Diabetes and fat are more likely to happen if your cells' metabolism isn't working right.
- *Neurodegenerative Diseases:* Alzheimer's and Parkinson's diseases cause cells to break down more quickly when you're under a lot of stress.

Chronic stress has effects on more than just mental health. It also has deep effects on cellular health and general health. Chronic worry can lead to a lot of different health problems because it speeds up aging, slows down repair processes, and makes inflammation worse. Getting rid of worry is important for more than just your mental health; it's also essential for the health and longevity of your cells.

Techniques for Reducing Stress: Mindfulness, Meditation, and Breathing

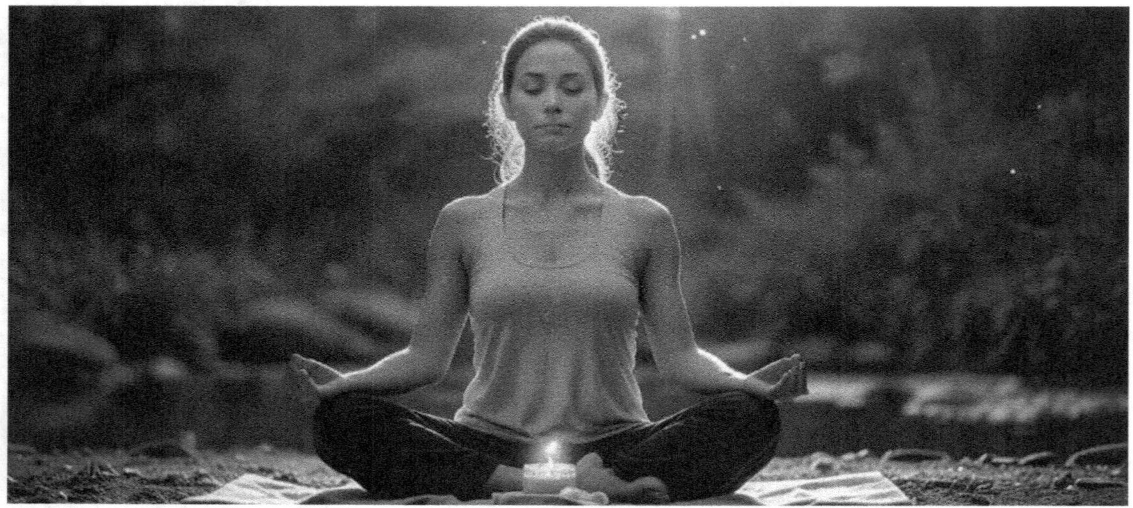

Managing stress well is important for keeping cells healthy and for your general health. Mindfulness, meditation, and breathing exercises are all powerful, scientifically proven ways to lower stress by calming the nervous system, making it easier to control your emotions, and making you stronger. These techniques help the body heal, renew, and stay healthy by reducing the negative effects of long-term stress, especially at the cellular level.

Mindfulness: Being in the Present Moment

What Does Mindfulness Mean?

Observing the present without judgment is mindfulness. To relax, pay attention to your thoughts, feelings, and surroundings.

How Mindfulness Supports Cellular Health

- *Lower Cortisol Levels:* Being mindful lowers the production of cortisol, which helps protect cells from the damage that long-term worry causes.
- *Longer telomeres:* Mindfulness can protect telomeres, which are the caps that cover DNA and slow down cellular aging, according to studies.
- *Improved immune function:* Regular mindfulness practice strengthens the immune system, aiding in cell recovery and defense.

How to Make Mindfulness a Habit

- For the body scan, lie down or sit down easily. Slowly focus on each part of your body, beginning with your toes and working your way up. Feel whatever is going on without judging it.
- *Mindful Eating:* Pay attention to how each bite tastes, feels, and smells. This not only lowers stress, but it also helps the body digest food and absorb nutrients.
- *Daily Awareness:* Bring awareness to things you do every day, like taking a walk, doing the dishes, or drinking tea. Pay attention to your feelings, actions, and movement.

Meditation: Getting Calm Inside

How do you Meditate?

Focusing your attention and getting rid of distractions are important parts of meditation, which helps you feel calm and clear-headed. Each type of meditation reduces stress differently.

How Meditation Supports Cellular Health

- *Lowers Oxidative Stress:* Meditation reduces the generation of reactive oxygen species (ROS), reducing the likelihood of oxidative stress damaging cells.
- *Enhances neuroplasticity:* regular meditation fosters the growth and repair of neurons, thereby promoting the health of brain cells and enhancing emotional regulation.
- *Maintains the equilibrium of the autonomic nervous system:* meditation activates the parasympathetic "rest-and-digest" system, counteracting the stress-induced fight-or-flight response.

Types of Meditation to Reduce Stress

- *Mindfulness meditation:* Pay attention to your breath or an object in the room and let your ideas come and go without judging them.
- *Kindness and love Practice meditation:* Repeat, "May I be happy and healthy," and wish the same for others to become more compassionate.
- *Guided Visualization:* Listen to a meditation that leads you to a peaceful place in your mind. This activity can lower cortisol levels and help you relax.

Tips on How to Begin Meditating

- Pick a quiet place and give yourself 5–10 minutes every day.
- Take a deep breath in and out, close your eyes, and focus on a phrase or your breath.

- Bring your attention back to the center point slowly if your mind wanders.
- As you become accustomed to the workouts, extend them gradually.

Breathing Techniques: Resetting the Nervous System

The Importance of Breathing

Breathing directly affects the parasympathetic nervous system. Deep, focused breathing tells the brain to calm down, which lowers stress hormones and makes you feel better.

How Breathing Supports Cellular Health

- *Boosts oxygen delivery:* Deep breathing enhances oxygenation, facilitating mitochondrial function and energy production.
- *Maintains proper pH levels:* Deep breathing regulates blood pH, ensuring optimal cell function.
- *Lessens inflammation:* Controlled breathing reduces inflammatory markers in the body, preventing stress-induced damage to cells.

Effective Breathing Techniques

Breathing through the diaphragm

- Hold out your arms and put one hand on your chest.
- Take a deep breath in through your nose, making sure your chest stays still and your belly rises.
- Let your belly fall as you slowly breathe out through your mouth.
- Practice for five to ten minutes to immediately feel less stressed.

Box Breathing

- Take four deep breaths in through your nose.
- Hold your breath for four counts.
- Breathe slowly through your mouth for four counts.

- Pause for four counts and then do it again.
- This method relaxes the mind and helps you concentrate.

Alternate Nostril Breathing

- Soak up some air, and close your right nostril with your thumb.
- Take a deep breath in through your left nose.
- Close the left nostril with your ring finger and let out air through the right one.
- Do this five times to balance your energy and calm down.

4. 4. 4–7 Breathing

- Take four deep breaths in through your nose.
- Do not breathe for seven seconds.
- Breathe out slowly through your mouth for eight seconds.
- This method works especially well for helping you sleep and relax.

Combining Techniques for Maximum Benefit

- *Mindful Breathing:* Focus on how each breath feels as it enters and leaves your body. This is a combination of awareness and deep breathing.
- *Meditative Movement:* Mindfulness, breathing, and slow movement are all part of yoga and tai chi, which makes stress relief even stronger.
- *Daily Rituals:* Spend a few minutes on at least one of these activities every day to help you deal with stress in a way that fits your lifestyle.

Mindfulness, meditation, and breathing movements are all beneficial ways to lower stress and keep cells healthy. They help you feel calmer, make you stronger, and protect cells from the damage that long-term worry can do. Doing these things daily can improve your mental and cell health, helping you live longer.

How to Integrate Stress Reduction into Your Daily Life

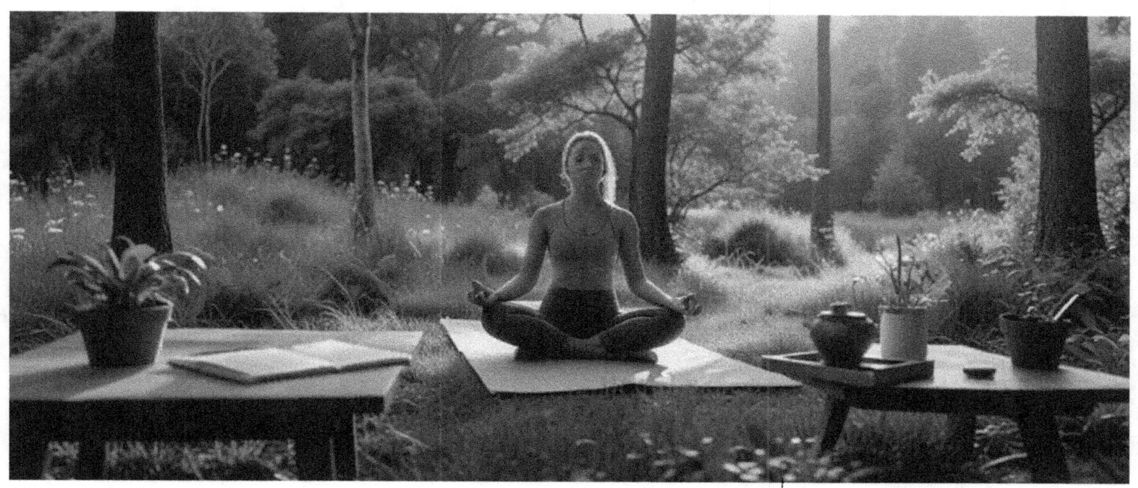

Relaxing once in a while isn't enough to lower your stress; you need to make it a habit to do things that are beneficial for your mental and physical health. If you want to truly protect your cells from the damage that long-term stress causes, you must manage your stress every day. Here are some useful tips that will help you easily incorporate techniques for reducing stress into your daily life.

Start Your Day with Intention

The way you start your day shapes how you deal with stress. Mindful practices can help you feel more grounded and ready to take on obstacles.

Stress Releasing Morning Routine

- *Mindful Breathing:* When you wake up, focus on your breath for five minutes using methods like diaphragmatic breathing or 4-7-8 breathing.
- *Keeping a journal:* To stay positive and on track, write down three things you're thankful for and your goals for the day.
- *Yoga or gentle stretches:* A short yoga routine or a few gentle stretches can loosen up your body, improve circulation, and get your mind ready for the day.

Benefits: These activities lower cortisol levels, make thinking clearer, and make it less likely that you will feel stressed.

Incorporate Mini Breaks into Your Day

Workdays with a lot of stress or busy plans can drain your energy and make you mentally tired. Taking breaks often helps you stay calm and get things done.

How to Take Breaks That Will Help You Relax:

- Use the Pomodoro Technique: work for 25 minutes, then take a 5-minute break to stretch, breathe deeply, or go outside and get some fresh air.
- Use mindfulness apps. For example, Calm or Headspace can help you do short exercises during breaks to get your mind back on track.
- Stress can make your muscles tense and then relax. Progressive muscle relaxation (PMR) is a way to ease the strain in your body.

Tip: Use your phone or calendar to tell yourself to take breaks, especially when things are busy or stressful.

Cultivate Stress-Reducing Rituals

Rituals give you order and predictability, which can help you deal with the stress of life's unknowns. These habits may seem easy, but they can be very relaxing.

Ideas for Daily Habits:

- *Tea Time:* Take 10 minutes to enjoy the warmth and smell of herbal tea, such as chamomile or green tea, with full attention.
- *End-of-Day Reflection:* Write in a gratitude book or think about the positive things that happened during the day for five minutes before bed.
- After dinner, a 15-minute walk can help your body digest food, clear your mind, and get ready for a wonderful night's sleep.

Pro Tip: Make these habits a must for you to consistently lower your stress.

Create an Environment that Helps you Deal with Stress.

Your environment has a big effect on how stressed you are. To stay calm throughout the day, making your surroundings more relaxing is helpful.

Changes to the Environment:

- *Clean up your space.* A place that is clean and well-organized helps you think more clearly and feel less stressed.
- *Bring Nature Inside:* To help you relax, add indoor plants or decor inspired by nature to your home or office.
- *Try aromatherapy.* Diffusing essential oils like lavender, peppermint, and sandalwood can help you feel less stressed and more relaxed.

Quick Tip: Change the lights in your space to include warm, natural tones. These tones are relaxing and less likely to make you feel stressed.

Prioritize Sleep and Rest

Getting enough rest is important for dealing with stress and keeping cells healthy. People who don't get enough sleep are more likely to have strong stress reactions and trouble dealing with worry.

How to Get a Better Night's Sleep:

- Setting up a relaxing routine before bed, like reading, breathing, or taking a warm bath, can help you wind down.
- *Make a sleep schedule.* Start going to bed and getting up at the same time every day, even on the weekends, to keep your circadian cycle in check.
- *Limit Screen Time:* To help your body make more melatonin, stay away from gadgets that give off blue light for at least an hour before bed.

Bonus Tip: To help you relax even more, try adding sleep-inducing teas or magnesium tablets (after talking to your doctor first).

Make Movement a Daily Habit.

One of the best ways to deal with worry is to do something active. Exercise releases endorphins, your body's natural mood boosters.

Ways to Include Movement:

- *Morning yoga or stretching:* Even 10 minutes of movement can wake you up and benefit you.
- *Active Commutes:* If you can, walk or ride a bike to work, or use the stairs instead of the lifts.
- *Dancing:* Play your best music and dance without stopping. It's a relaxing way to get rid of stress and burn calories.

Move in a way that you enjoy to make it a practice instead of something you have to do.

Talk to Other People

Social interactions reduce stress by fostering a sense of belonging and support. Oxytocin is a hormone that fights stress hormones like cortisol. Good relationships release this hormone.

How to Stay Connected:

- *Make time for people you care about:* Call or meet up with friends and family often, even if it's just for a short chat.
- *Join groups:* Attend community events, exercise classes, or support groups to meet new people and share your stories.
- *Show Gratitude:* Being thankful for the people in your life makes your relationships stronger and makes you feel better.

Pro Tip: To avoid burnout, find a mix between socializing and taking time to relax.

Think Positively and Show Gratitude.

Changing the way you think can greatly lower stress. Recognizing the positive things in your life can change how you deal with problems and worry.

Daily Gratitude Practices:

- Every day, write down three things you're grateful for.
- To end the day on a positive note, think about the positive things that happened to you before bed.
- Say affirmations to yourself every day, like "I can handle problems with calm and grace."

Bonus Tip: For an even stronger way to reduce stress, combine being grateful with being aware.

Use Technology to Support Stress Reduction

Technology can stress you out, but uses it wisely can be helpful.

Apps that can help you deal with stress:

- Headspace or Calm offer guided meditations and breathing routines.
- *Forest:* It helps you focus by reducing internet distractions.
- *MyFitnessPal or Fitbit:* Tracks your sleep, awareness, and movement for a more comprehensive view of your health.

Avoid excessive screen time as it can lead to stress. Set limits on your apps.

Be Steady and Patient.

Getting into beneficial habits takes time, and dealing with stress well needs a slow, steady approach. Allow yourself some time as you start to include these things in your daily life.

Big Changes from Small Steps:

- Begin with a few skills and add to them as you go.
- Think about what works once a week and make changes as needed.
- Celebrate small wins to keep going.

Getting rid of stress in your daily life isn't just about doing a few things here and there; it's about making a whole, helpful lifestyle. You can better handle stress, protect your cell health, and promote long-term vitality by making awareness, movement, connection, and gratitude a regular part of your life. Making small changes over time can have big effects, enabling you to live a more peaceful and strong life.

CHAPTER 11

ENVIRONMENTAL FACTORS – PROTECTING YOUR CELLS FROM EXTERNAL STRESSORS

The world around us has a huge effect on the health of our cells. The chemicals in everyday items and the air we breathe constantly stress our cells, preventing them from functioning optimally. This chapter talks about the main external factors that can hurt cell health, suggests ways to reduce these effects, and gives useful advice on how to make a safe and healthy place to live.

The Impact of Pollution, EMFs, and Toxins on Cellular Health

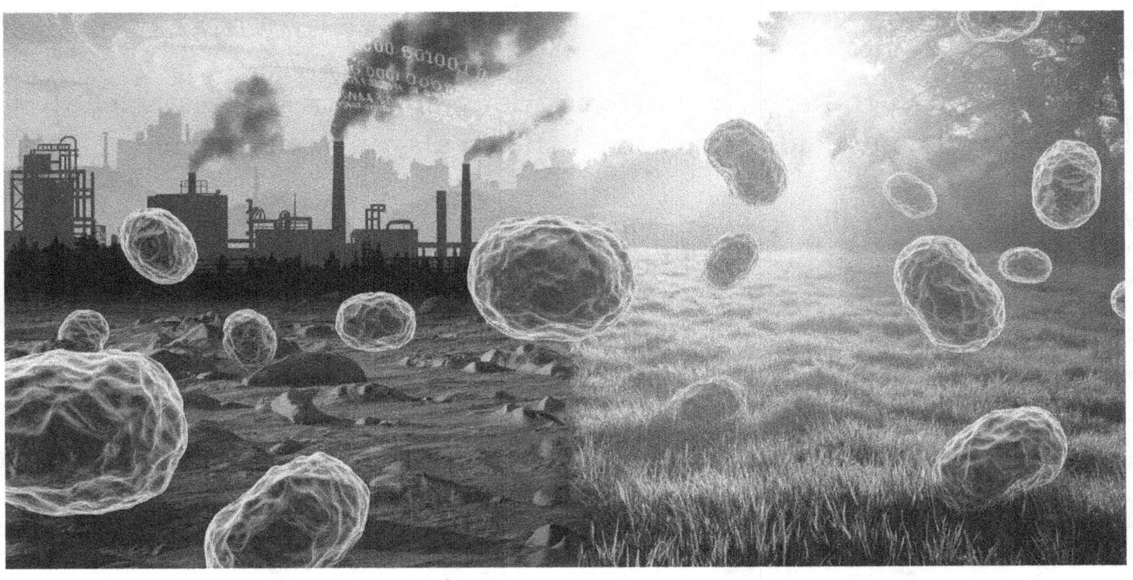

Toxins, electromagnetic fields (EMFs), pollution, and other things in the environment are dangerous for cell health. These outside stresses can mess up normal cellular processes, add to oxidative stress, and speed up the aging process. Knowing how they affect us gives us the power to protect our cells and limit our exposure.

Pollution and Cellular Damage

Air Pollution

Air pollution is a big problem for the environment. Pollutants like carbon monoxide, ozone, nitrogen dioxide (NO_2), and fine particulate matter (PM2.5) are very common. These tiny particles and gases enter the body through the lungs, entering the bloodstream and all cells.

- *Oxidative Stress:* Pollutants make reactive oxygen species (ROS), which hurt DNA, proteins, and lipids inside cells.
- *Inflammation:* Long-term contact causes systemic inflammation, which makes it harder for cells to heal themselves.
- *Aging and Disease:* Long-term exposure to polluted air is associated with faster aging, breathing issues, heart disease, and even illnesses that damage nerve cells.

Water Pollution

Polluted water contains a variety of dangerous substances, including heavy metals, pesticides, industrial chemicals, and pathogens.

- *Heavy Metals:* Arsenic, lead, and mercury mess up the way cells talk to each other and how mitochondria work, which can lead to neurotoxicity and metabolic diseases.
- *Pesticides and Industrial Chemicals*: Persistent organic pollutants (POPs) build up in fatty tissues, making it harder for cells to get rid of toxins and raising the risk of cancer.

Indoor Pollution

Home goods like paints, cleaners, and furniture often contain volatile organic compounds (VOCs).

- *Toxic Exposure:* When VOCs contact the skin or enter the lungs, they damage DNA and cellular membranes.
- *Long-Term Conditions:* Prolonged exposure is associated with asthma, allergies, and other inflammatory conditions.

Electromagnetic Fields (EMFs) and Cellular Health

Electronic items like microwaves, smartphones, and Wi-Fi routers send out electromagnetic fields. While low levels of electromagnetic fields (EMF) are considered safe, prolonged exposure to high levels can disrupt the functioning of cells.

- *Calcium Channel Disruption:* EMFs can open voltage-gated calcium channels, which lets too much calcium into cells. This leads to reactive stress and stops cells from communicating normally.
- *Dysfunction of the mitochondria: The* powerhouses of cells, mitochondria, are particularly sensitive to stress from electromagnetic fields (EMFs), which causes them to produce less energy and more reactive oxygen species.
- *Damage to DNA:* Some studies show that long-term exposure to EMFs may break DNA strands, which raises the risk of mutations and cancer.

Toxins in Everyday Products

Another major contributor to cellular stress is the presence of chemicals in many personal care and home items.

Phthalates and Parabens

- Plastic items, cosmetics, and shampoos all contain it.
- Effects on cells: These chemicals interfere with hormones and disrupt normal cell communication, which can negatively impact sexual health.

Bisphenol A (BPA)

- *Sources:* The linings of food cans and plastic containers commonly contain this substance.
- *Effects on cells:* BPA disrupts the function of mitochondria and DNA repair, which can result in metabolic issues and chronic inflammation

Pesticides

- Residues on non-organic food are the sources.
- Effects on cells: Pesticides stop cellular detoxification enzymes from working, which makes it harder for cells to get rid of dangerous substances.

Heavy Metals

- It is present in fish, industrial waste, and contaminated water.
- Effects on cells: Heavy metals mess up the way enzymes work, hurt DNA, and add to oxidative stress.

The Long-Term Effects of Environmental Stressors

Oxidative Stress

Toxins and pollutants in the environment make ROS, which causes a state known as oxidative stress. Because ROS and the body's antioxidant protections are out of balance,

- Cellular Aging: The protective caps on chromosomes called telomeres are shortening faster.
- For example, arthritis, heart disease, and diabetes are all inflammatory diseases.
- DNA abnormalities increase the risk of cancer.

Disruption of cellular energy

EMFs and pollutants make mitochondrial function worse, which lowers the production of ATP (energy). This makes you tired, lowers your immune system, and makes it challenging for your cells to heal.

Hormonal Imbalance

Toxins like BPA and phthalates mess up the way endocrine systems work, which makes it challenging for hormones to work properly. This can have an effect on your metabolism, growth, and ability to have children.

Weakening of the Immune System

Exposure to external stressors weakens the immune system over time. This makes the body more likely to get infections and slows the healing of wounds.

Pollution, electromagnetic fields (EMFs), and chemicals can damage cells, which is why we need to take action to protect our health. Even though we can't completely avoid these environmental stresses, there are things we can do to lessen their effects. Some of these include choosing non-toxic products, cleaning the air and water, and reducing your exposure to electromagnetic fields (EMFs). By doing these things, we can keep our cells healthy and improve our general health.

How to Minimize Environmental Harm to Your Cells

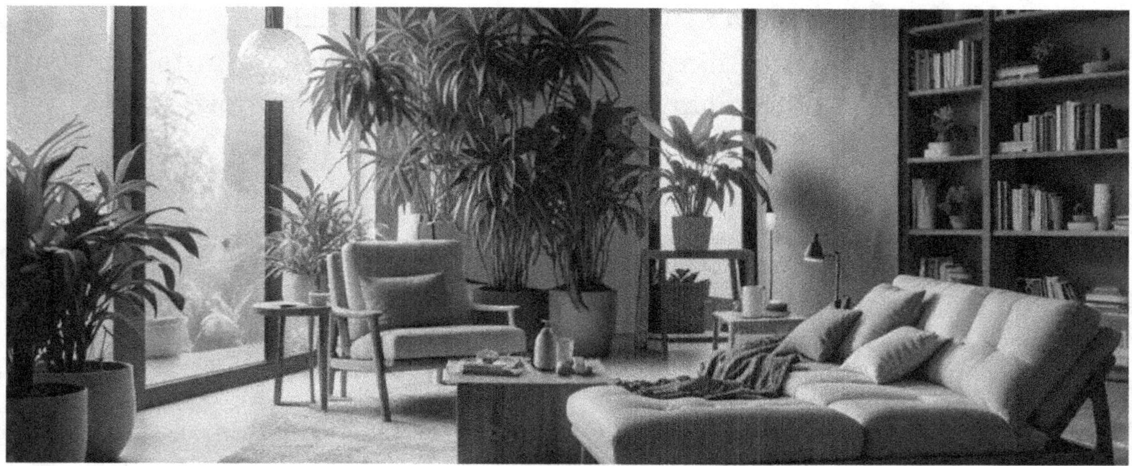

To protect cellular health, it is important to limit exposure to environmental factors like pollution, electromagnetic fields (EMFs), and toxins. Avoiding them completely is not possible, but being proactive can greatly reduce their harmful effects and help cells stay strong. Here are some useful ways to keep your cells safe.

Reducing Exposure to Air Pollution

Indoor Air Quality

- Use air purifiers. To get rid of small particles, allergens, and pollutants in your home, buy high-quality air purifiers with HEPA filters.
- Let air flow through: Make sure there is adequate air flow by regularly opening windows or using ventilation systems, especially when you are cooking or cleaning.
- Stay away from indoor pollutants. For example, don't use too many air fresheners, candles, or perfumes that give off volatile organic compounds (VOCs).

Outdoor Air Quality

- *Keep an eye on pollution levels.* There are apps and websites that can help you keep track of air quality levels in your area. If pollution levels are high, don't go outside.
- *Make a Wall:* If you're walking in a city, stay away from places with a lot of traffic. If pollution levels are always high, you might want to wear a mask that filters out fine particles.
- Add more plants, like peace flowers or snake plants, to your home. These plants can help clean the air and remove toxins.

Limiting Toxins in Water

- Use a Water Filter: To get rid of heavy metals, chlorine, and other contaminants, put in a reputable water filter system. Select water filters that have undergone testing and proven to eliminate specific contaminants.
- Drink from glass or stainless steel. Plastic bottles, particularly those that have been exposed to heat, can leach harmful chemicals such as BPA into the water.
- Test Your Water Supply: Check your tap water often for contaminants and pick the right ways to filter it.

Choose Safer Personal Care and Home Goods

Self-Care

- *Read the labels:* Stay away from items that have parabens, phthalates, triclosan, or artificial fragrances in them. Look for beauty names that are clean and don't add a lot of chemicals.
- *Choose natural alternatives:* To limit your exposure to chemicals, use homemade or organic hair and skin care products.

Household Cleaners

- Use cleaners that are better for the environment. Instead of regular cleaners, use ones made from natural ingredients like citric acid, baking soda, or vinegar.
- Don't use too many herbicides and pesticides. If you do have to use them, be sure to follow all safety rules and wear protection gear.

Reducing Exposure to Electromagnetic Fields (EMFs)

- *Turn Off Devices:* To avoid extra EMF radiation, turn off electronics like Wi-Fi routers and smartphones at night.
- *Use wired connections:* Ethernet cords are better than Wi-Fi, and wired headphones are better than Bluetooth headphones when you can.
- *Keep a Safe Distance:* Stay away from sources of EMF. For example, don't sleep with your phone close to your head or use a laptop on your lap.
- *Spend money on shielding.* Cases, paint, and fabrics that block EMFs can help you stay safe in high-EMF places.

Eating A Healthy, Non-Toxic Diet

- *Choose Organic Produce:* To avoid getting too much pesticide residue on your food, choose organic fruits and veggies, especially those on the "Dirty Dozen" list.
- *Wash very well:* To get rid of pesticides, use a vegetable wash or soak fruits and vegetables in water with baking soda.

- *Stay away from processed foods.* Packaged and processed foods often have colors, additives, and preservatives that stress the body's detoxification pathways.

Supporting Cellular Detoxification

- *Drink a lot of water.* Staying hydrated helps the kidneys work better and gets rid of waste from the body.
- *Eat Foods High in Fiber:* Leafy greens, beans, and whole grains are all high in fiber and help the body get rid of toxins.
- *Eat foods that help the liver detox.* For example, cruciferous veggies (broccoli, kale, cauliflower) and garlic are beneficial examples of foods that help the liver detox.
- *Be Smart About Supplements:* If you want to use milk thistle, N-acetyl cysteine (NAC), or activated charcoal as supplements to help your body clean, talk to your doctor first.

Creating an environment conducive to cell growth

Reduce Indoor Toxins

- *Get rid of products that give off VOCs.* You should stay away from furniture, rugs, and paints that do this. Pick water-based options that are safe.
- *Lower the humidity:* To stop mold growth, which can release mycotoxins that are detrimental for cell health, use a dehumidifier.
- *Clear out your space:* A clean, well-organized home needs fewer strong cleaning products and less dust buildup.

Sleep and Relax in Clean Spaces

- *Buy a quality mattress.* To stay away from flame retardants and synthetic materials, use organic beds and bedding that are free of chemicals.
- *Sleep with Clean Air:* To sleep in a toxin-free space, use an air filter in your bedroom.

Supporting Resilience Through Lifestyle Choices

- Work out regularly. Exercise improves circulation, which helps cells get oxygen and nutrients and speeds up the removal of cellular waste.
- Practice mindful breathing. Deep, controlled breathing can lower oxidative stress and help cells get more oxygen.
- Spend time in nature. Being outside, especially in green places, can help you feel less stressed and breathe better.

Advocate for Environmental Changes

- Support green projects by advocating for laws that reduce smog and promote clean energy.
- *Teach Others:* Tell others what you know about how natural toxins affect people and how to protect themselves from them.
- *Cut down on waste:* participate in recycling programs and use less single-use plastic to help protect the earth.

To keep environmental damage to your cells to a minimum, you should limit your exposure to chemicals, live a clean lifestyle, and make your home toxin-free. These steps will not only protect the health of your cells, but they will also improve your general health and vitality. Consider that even small changes over time can have big impacts on your health and the world.

Creating a Healthy, Cell-Friendly Living Environment

Your home and workplace have a big effect on the health of your cells. Your cells can work at their best when they are in a clean, toxin-free, and balanced atmosphere. Creating a cell-friendly place means lowering exposure to harmful substances, making the air and water cleaner, and improving the environment as a whole to help cells heal and stay healthy.

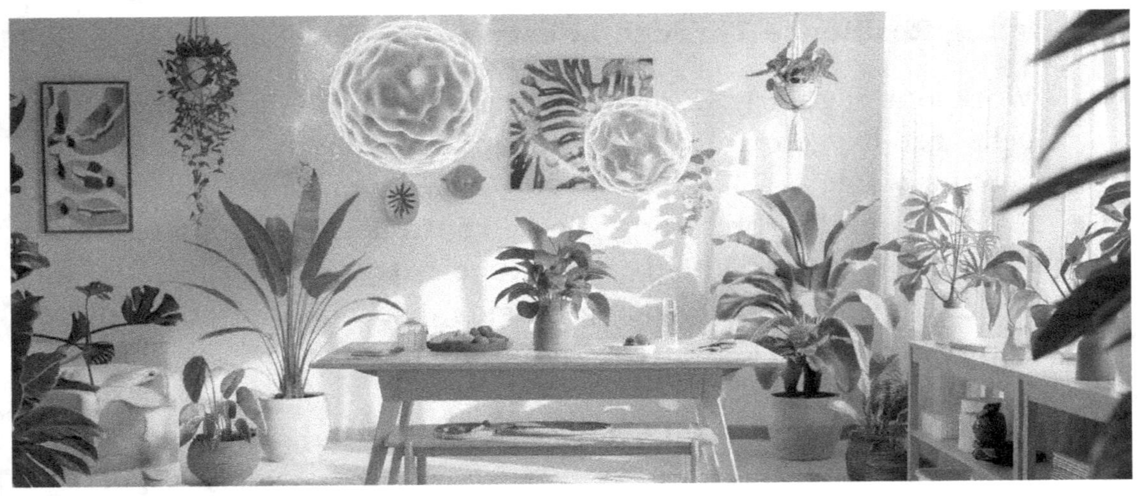

Making the Air Quality Better

Air Inside

- Use air purifiers. A high-efficiency particulate air (HEPA) filter gets rid of dust, allergens, and pollutants in the air, which is beneficial for your lungs and gives cells more oxygen.
- Make sure there is enough airflow by opening windows often to let fresh air in. To lower the amount of pollution and humidity inside, use vent fans in the kitchen and bathroom.
- Use houseplants. Spider plants, peace lilies, and Boston ferns are some examples of plants that help clean the air inside and remove toxins like formaldehyde and benzene.

Outside Air

- Make a green wall around your house by planting trees or bushes to block out noise and pollution. These natural barriers make the air better and create a calm space.

Improving Water Quality

- *Put in water filters.* To get rid of dangerous substances like chlorine, lead, and heavy metals, use activated carbon or reverse osmosis filters.

- *Don't use plastic bottles.* Instead, use stainless steel or glass bottles so that chemicals don't get into your water.
- *Regular Maintenance*: To make sure that the toxin removal works well, clean and change the filters as needed.

Monitor electromagnetic and light exposure

Natural Light

- Get the most daylight: Keep your windows open during the day to let natural light into your home. Natural light helps your circadian rhythm and keeps your cell repair processes healthy.
- Add full-spectrum lighting. If there isn't a lot of natural light in a room, use full-spectrum bulbs that look like sunlight to keep the room balanced.

Minimizing EMFs

- Keep electronics away: Keep electronics like computers, smartphones, and routers away from places where you sleep to lower your electromagnetic field (EMF) exposure while you sleep.
- Turn Off Devices: At night, unplug electronics that you don't need and turn off Wi-Fi routers.
- Use EMF Shields: To protect yourself from too much contact, buy cases, fabrics, or paints that lower EMFs.

Limiting Toxins in the Home

Products for Personal Care

- Use natural goods instead. Shampoos, soaps, and skin care items that don't contain artificial scents, parabens, or phthalates are better for you. Choose items that say they are organic or not toxic on the box.

Cleaning Products

- *Do It Yourself Cleaners:* Using vinegar, baking soda, and lemon juice together, you can make simple cleaning products that work well and are safe for you and the environment.
- *Pick green brands:* Look for cleaning goods that are safe for the environment and have eco-friendly labels.

Enhancing Sleeping Spaces

The Bedroom Setting

- Use organic bedding. To avoid flame retardants and synthetic chemicals, switch to beds, pillows, and sheets made from natural materials like wool or organic cotton that are free of chemicals.
- Get rid of the junk in your bedroom. A clean and organized space helps you relax and lowers stress, germs, and dust.

Temperature for Sleeping

- Keep yourself comfortable: Keep your bedroom cool (18–22°C or 65–72°F) to help you get long, restorative sleep, which is important for fixing cells.

Reducing Noise Pollution

- Keep noise out of the room by using thick curtains, rugs, or acoustic walls.
- Make quiet areas: Set aside places that are free of noise and other distractions where you can relax or meditate.

Balancing Humidity Levels

- Stop Mold Growth: Use dehumidifiers or air conditioners to keep the humidity level between 30 and 50% to stop mold, which can release dangerous mycotoxins.
- Monitor the humidity levels in your home using hygrometers to ensure they remain within a healthy range.

Adding Natural Elements

- Wood and stone: Purchase furniture and home decor made from untreated natural materials to reduce your chemical exposure.
- Biophilic Design: Use designs, textures, and colors that come from nature to make your home more relaxing and beneficial for your cells.

Maintaining your Mental and Emotional Well-Being

Calming Spaces

- Make relaxation corners. These are areas designed for relaxation or meditation, featuring soft lighting, comfortable seating, and natural elements.
- Aromatherapy: Put lavender or eucalyptus essential oils in diffusers to make the room feel calm and relaxing and to lower your stress.

Minimize Digital Overload

- Setting up screen-free places in your home can help your mind feel less fatigued and your cells recover faster.

Making sure the Space is Clean and Organized

- Regularly get rid of clutter: a clean space makes you feel better and keeps dust and other pollution from building up.
- Deep Clean Once in a While: For regular cleaning, use non-toxic cleaners, and once in a while, clean places that get dirty easily, like vents and rugs.

Supporting Your Lifestyle

- Ergonomic Design: Set up work areas so that they lower physical stress and improve posture, which increases blood flow and cellular energy.
- Green Outdoor Areas: Spend time in nature to get fresh air, sunlight, and surroundings that help you relax.

Making changes to the surroundings in a way that is beneficial for cells means getting rid of toxins, making the water and air cleaner, and making the lighting and sound better. By focusing on natural elements, limiting exposure to harmful substances, and keeping your space clean and organized, you build a foundation for healthy cells, long life, and general well-being.

PART 4:

BUILDING RESILIENCE AT THE CELLULAR LEVEL

CHAPTER 12

IMMUNE SYSTEM SUPPORT – STRENGTHENING YOUR CELLS AGAINST DISEASE

Your immune system is the first line of defense against germs, illnesses, and other outside threats. It works with your cells and depends on their health and efficiency to make a strong defense against threats. Increasing the strength of your cells directly boosts your immune system, making your body stronger so it can fight off illness and stay healthy.

How Cellular Health and Immunity Are Interconnected

The immune system needs cells that are healthy and working well to keep the body safe from pathogens, fix harmed tissues, and keep everyone healthy. Cells form the foundation of the immune response, and the health of these cells directly influences the effectiveness and duration of the immune response. Understanding the link between these two factors can enhance your understanding of how your food, lifestyle, and environment can support the optimal functioning of your immune system.

Cellular Function as the Foundation of Immunity

There are different types of immune cells, like leukocytes, T-cells, B-cells, and macrophages, which are white blood cells. These cells perform various tasks such as identifying, halting, and eliminating harmful invaders such as bacteria, viruses, and toxins. In order to do these things, immune cells need to be fully effective, which depends on

- *Making energy:* Cells need enough energy to fight off bugs and start their defenses. The energy centers of cells, called mitochondria, are crucial for immune reactions.

- *Signal Transmission:* Chemical messengers, like cytokines, help healthy cells talk to each other. They organize the immune system's attack and repair plans.
- *Cell Renewal and Repair:* Immune cells are always dividing and renewing to keep their numbers and abilities up. Cellular health makes sure that these processes go smoothly.

The Role of Mitochondria in Immune Response

Mitochondria are crucial for keeping the defense system going. ATP is the energy currency that cells use to do their jobs. These tiny organelles make it. It takes a lot more energy for immune cells to do their job when they are active, like when they are fighting an infection.

- *Energy and Activation:* Immune cells need energy to multiply quickly and efficiently, and healthy mitochondria give them that energy.
- *Reactive Oxygen Species (ROS):* Mitochondria not only make energy, but they also make ROS, which are chemicals that help immune cells kill pathogens. However, an excess of ROS can harm healthy cells, underscoring the significance of striking a balance between energy production and antioxidant-based cell protection.

Oxidative Stress and Cell Damage

Free radicals (like ROS) and the body's antioxidant protections are out of balance, which leads to oxidative stress. Because they work in places with lots of free radicals during immune responses, immune cells are especially sensitive to oxidative stress.

- *Effects on Immune Cells:* Too much oxidative stress can hurt the DNA, proteins, and membranes of immune cells, making them less able to do their job.
- *Cellular Health Link:* Antioxidants, like vitamin C, vitamin E, and selenium, found in a healthy diet, protect cells from toxic damage, which keeps the immune system working well.

Chronic Inflammation and Immune Dysregulation

Inflammation that lasts for a long time, called chronic inflammation, can put stress on the health of cells. To heal and protect, acute inflammation is essential. But long-term inflammation causes:

- *Immune Fatigue:* Overworked immune cells may lose their effectiveness, making it more difficult for them to fight infections or heal tissues.
- *Damage to tissue and cells:* Long-term inflammation can hurt cells around it, starting a cycle of damage and repair that makes the immune system less strong overall. By making anti-inflammatory molecules and keeping the structure of the tissue, healthy cells are better able to reduce inflammation.

The Gut-Immune Axis and Cellular Health

The gut is home to about 70% of the immune system. There, immune cells interact with the gut microbiome, which is a population of trillions of microorganisms. It is in the gut that immune cells learn how to tell the difference between dangerous invaders and helpful substances.

- *Nutrient Absorption:* Enterocytes, healthy intestinal cells, ensure the absorption of vital nutrients that support immune cell growth and repair.
- Pathogens and toxins can't get into the bloodstream when the gut lining is strong. This makes the immune system's job easier.
- *Microbiome Balance:* Good bacteria in the gut make substances called short-chain fatty acids (SCFAs) that help immune cells work better and lower inflammation.

Cellular Communication in Immunity

Immune cells need to be able to talk to each other clearly in order to organize their responses. Signaling molecules like cytokines and chemokines help immune cells find and attack attackers more effectively.

- *Healthy Cell Membranes:* When cellular membranes contain healthy fats like omega-3s, signaling pathways function more effectively.
- *Dependence on Nutrients:* Some of the nutrients required to produce and regulate these communication molecules include zinc, magnesium, and vitamin D.

Cellular Renewal and Immune Defense

A steady flow of new, healthy cells is important for the defense system. The bone marrow, which produces the defense cells, requires iron, folate, and vitamin B12 for hematopoiesis, the process of producing blood cells.

- *Immunity and Stem Cells:* In the bone marrow, stem cells change into different types of immunity cells. Cellular health makes sure that these stem cells can work well and divide properly.
- *Autophagy:* This natural process helps cells get rid of broken parts, which lowers the risk of cells not working right and keeps the immune system strong.

Lifestyle Factors Linking Cellular and Immune Health

Certain habits directly impact the health of cells and, consequently, the immune system.

- *Nutrition:* Insufficient nutrients can hinder the production and function of immune cells.
- *Hydration:* Water makes it easier for trash and nutrients to move in and out of cells.
- *Exercise:* Being active improves circulation, which helps immune cells get more air and nutrients.
- *Sleep:* Deep sleep aids in the healing of cells and the growth of new defense cells.
- *Managing stress:* Long-term stress messes up the way cells work, which makes the immune system weaker.

There is a direct link between the defense system and the health of cells. Strong immunity saves cells from damage and disease, and healthy cells help the immune system work well. Prioritizing a nutrient-dense diet, dealing with stress, keeping hydrated, and forming healing habits can improve the health of your cells and immune system, making you less likely to get sick and promoting long-term vitality.

What to Eat and Take to Boost Your Immunity

A strong immune system needs a steady flow of nutrients that keep cells healthy and help immune cells do their job. Certain foods and supplements contribute significantly to your overall health by providing essential vitamins, minerals, antioxidants, and bioactive substances. Adding these to your diet can help your immune system work better and keep you from getting sick.

Foods High in Nutrients to Help the Immune System

The best foods for your immune system are those that are high in antioxidants, herbs, vitamins, and minerals. These nutrients enhance cell function and prevent damage to immune cells.

Fruits and Vegetables

- Citrus foods, like oranges, lemons, and grapefruits, are high in vitamin C, which helps the immune system work better and makes white blood cells grow.
- Antioxidants such as anthocyanins, found in berries like blueberries, strawberries, and raspberries, protect cells from oxidative stress.
- Leafy greens like spinach, kale, and Swiss chard are high in vitamins A and C, folate, and beta-carotene, all of which help defense cells stay healthy and heal.
- Cruciferous vegetables, like broccoli, Brussels sprouts, and cauliflower, have sulforaphane in them, a chemical that helps the immune system and boosts cleansing enzymes.

- Carrots and sweet potatoes: They contain beta-carotene, which is a building block for vitamin A and helps the skin's defense against germs.

Protein Sources

- Lean meats like chicken, turkey, and fish provide zinc, a mineral that is important for the growth and coordination of immune cells.
- Foods that are high in plant-based proteins, iron, and zinc are legumes (like lentils, chickpeas, and black beans).
- Eggs contain omega-3 fatty acids and vitamin D, which support your immune system.

Whole Grains

- Quinoa, brown rice, and oats: These foods provide immune cells with energy and are rich in B vitamins, essential for cell growth and repair.

Seeds and Nuts

- Sunflower, almond, and walnut seeds are rich in vitamin E, a potent antioxidant that combats free radicals and safeguards immune cells.

Healthy Fats

- Avocado, olive oil, and fatty fish like salmon and mackerel: These foods contain omega-3 fatty acids, which help the immune system and lower inflammation.

Probiotic-Rich Foods

- Yogurt (with live cultures), kimchi, sauerkraut, and kombucha all have good bacteria in them that improve gut health. This is important because 70% of the defense system is located in the gut.

Spices and Herbs

- Garlic has allicin in it, which is an antimicrobial substance that makes the immune system stronger.
- Turmeric contains a significant amount of curcumin, an anti-inflammatory chemical that aids in regulating the functioning of the immune system.
- Ginger: It has gingerol in it, which is an antioxidant and an anti-inflammatory.

Supplements that Boost the Immune System

A well-balanced diet is the best way to get all the nutrients you need, but some pills can help fill in the gaps or give your immune system extra support, especially when you are sick or under a lot of stress.

Vitamins

- For example, vitamin C helps defense cells grow and do their job. Ascorbic acid vitamins and foods like acerola cherries are both excellent sources of this acid.
- Vitamin D: It regulates the immune system and reduces the likelihood of illness. Supplements and being out in the sun are beneficial options.
- Vitamin A strengthens the skin and mucus membranes, which are the body's first line of defense against germs. Minerals

Minerals

- Zinc is essential for the growth and activity of immune cells like T-cells. You can find it in pills or lozenges.
- Selenium: It helps the body make immune proteins and vitamins. Brazil nuts and vitamins are good sources of selenium.
- Magnesium: helps the body make energy and lowers inflammation, which has a secondary effect on the immune system.

Antioxidants

- As the "master antioxidant," glutathione helps the body get rid of toxins and protects defense cells.
- Coenzyme Q10 (CoQ10): Aids in the production of energy within cells and provides protection against free radicals.

Probiotics

- Lactobacillus and Bifidobacterium Strains: These strains help the gut stay healthy, boost the immune system, and stop dangerous pathogens from taking over the digestive system.

Herbal Supplements

- It is known that elderberry extract can fight viruses and shorten the length of colds.
- Echinacea: This herb may make white blood cells work better and make colds last shorter.
- Astragalus Root: It enhances the function of the immune system and combats fatigue.

Hydration and Immunity

For the defense system to work properly, you need to stay hydrated. Water helps get rid of waste and boosts the body's defense system. It also helps nutrients and oxygen get to all parts of the body.

- Fluids High in Electrolytes: Coconut water or oral rehydration products help you stay hydrated and replace minerals that you've lost.
- Herbal Teas: Peppermint, chamomile, and green tea are all soothing and contain vitamins.

Here are Some Healthy Meal Ideas to Boost your Immune System.

Breakfast

- ***Immune-Boosting Smoothie:*** *Blend spinach, frozen berries, Greek yogurt, orange juice, and a teaspoon of turmeric.*

- ***Avocado Toast:*** *Whole-grain bread topped with mashed avocado, a poached egg, and a sprinkle of sunflower seeds.*

Lunch

- ***Quinoa Salad:*** *Toss cooked quinoa with chickpeas, cherry tomatoes, cucumber, olive oil, and lemon juice.*

- ***Garlic and Ginger Soup:*** *Bone broth with garlic, ginger, and shredded chicken for a warming, nutrient-rich meal.*

Dinner

- ***Baked Salmon with Sweet Potatoes:*** *Pair with a side of steamed broccoli or a leafy green salad.*

- ***Vegetable Stir-Fry:*** *Combine tofu, bell peppers, carrots, and onions with a turmeric-ginger sauce.*

Snacks

- ***Mixed Nuts and Seeds:*** *Almonds, walnuts, and pumpkin seeds.*

- ***Yogurt Parfait:*** *Layer plain yogurt with fresh berries and a drizzle of honey.*

Practical Tips for Maximizing Immune Benefits

- Select Whole Foods: To maintain their nutritional density, opt for foods with minimal processing.
- Eat a variety of fruits, veggies, and protein sources to get a full range of nutrients.

- Stay away from too much sugar and alcohol. Both can weaken your immune system and make inflammation worse.
- Timing your meals is important because immune cells need a steady source of energy.

By eating and taking vitamins that boost your immune system every day, you can make your body's defenses stronger against illness and improve the health of your cells. This well-balanced method includes eating foods that are high in nutrients, taking specific vitamins, and making changes to your lifestyle to keep your immune system strong for long-term health.

Lifestyle Habits for a Strong Immune System

Good eating alone doesn't guarantee a strong immune system; your lifelong habits also play a crucial role. By doing certain things, you can make it easier for your immune system to work well, lower your stress levels, and make yourself less likely to get sick.

Make Good Sleep a Priority.

- *Restorative Rest:* When you get deep sleep, your body makes molecules like cytokines that fight infections. Not getting enough sleep can weaken your immune system and make you more likely to get sick.
- *Regular Sleep Schedule:* Going to bed and getting up at the same time every day keeps the body's circadian cycle in balance, which is important for the immune system to work well.
- *Good sleep hygiene:* Make sure your bedroom is cool, dark, and quiet. To help your body make more melatonin, stay away from screens at least an hour before bed.

Learn How to Deal with Stress Well.

Chronic stress and immunity: Long-term stress increases cortisol levels, which can impair immunity. Keeping your immune system in balance requires that you deal with stress.

Daily Activities That Lower Stress: Ten to twenty minutes of mindfulness or meditation can help you rest. Engage in deep breathing exercises to reduce stress levels and soothe your thoughts. Take frequent breaks during your work to prevent your mind from becoming fatigued and stress from building up.

Keep up your Regular Exercise.

The benefits of moderate exercise: regular moderate-intensity exercise helps lymphatic flow, makes it easier for immune cells to move around, and lowers inflammation.

Regular Hints and Tips: Aim for 150 minutes of moderate exercise a week. Some examples of this would be yoga, cycling, or brisk walks. Engage in resistance training twice a week to maintain the health of your muscles and a healthy metabolism. Don't overtrain, because too much physical stress can briefly lower your immune system's ability to fight off sickness.

Drink Enough Water.

Water and Immunity: Maintaining hydration facilitates the transportation of nutrients and immunity cells, as well as the elimination of toxins.

Ways to keep drinking water: Drink a glass of water first thing in the morning to recover after sleeping. Putting cucumber or lemon slices in water makes it taste better and helps your immune system. Make sure you stay hydrated by checking your urine throughout the day to make sure it stays light yellow.

Improve your Gut Health

Gut-Immune Connection: About 70% of the immune system is located in the gut. To have a strong immune system, your gut bacteria need to be in balance.

Habits that help: Eat foods that are high in probiotics, like yogurt, kimchi, and kefir. Eat foods that are high in prebiotics, like garlic, onions, and asparagus, to keep beneficial bugs healthy. Do not take too many medicines unless your doctor tells you to. They can change the microbiota in your gut.

Spend Time Outside

Making vitamin D: Being in the sun helps the body make vitamin D, which is an important nutrient for optimal health.

The stress-relieving effect of nature: spending time in green areas lowers stress hormones and improves happiness, which indirectly helps the immune system.

Words of advice: Aim for 10 to 30 minutes of sunlight every day, but this will depend on your skin tone and where you live. As part of your weekly schedule, do things outside like hikes or gardening.

Maintain Strong Social Connections

Strong social ties and immunity: Research has shown that people with strong social ties are less likely to get sick. Having conversations with other people lowers stress and improves mental health.

Ways to Make Connections Stronger: Set up regular times to call or meet up with family and friends. Join clubs or neighborhood groups to feel like you belong. Do beneficial things for other people. It will improve your mood and strengthen your immune system.

Minimize Toxins and Pollutants

Environmental Risks: Pollutants in the air, smoking, and drinking too much alcohol can weaken defense cells and raise oxidative stress.

Good alternatives for health: Avoid smoking and secondhand smoke as they can weaken your lungs. We recommend moderate alcohol use, with women having one drink per day and men having two. To make the air in your home better, use air filters or houseplants.

Keep your Weight in a Healthy Range.

Being overweight can cause low-grade inflammation that lasts for a long time, which lowers the immune system's ability to fight off infections.

Sustainable Habits: Focus on whole, nutrient-dense foods and stay away from processed, high-sugar foods. To keep your metabolism healthy, do a lot of physical exercise and think about what you eat.

Engage in Regular Preventive Health Measures

Ensure you receive all recommended vaccines on time to maintain your health and prevent preventable diseases.

Good hygiene habits: Use soap and water to wash your hands often, especially before meals and after going to the bathroom. Avoid touching your face, particularly your eyes, nose, and mouth, to prevent the entry of pathogens.

Try to Keep a Positive Attitude.

Mental Health and Immunity: Studies have linked optimism and positive thinking to a stronger immune system and less inflammation from stress.

Ways to change your mind: Write down the positive things that happen in your life in a gratitude book. Visualization or mantras can boost resilience and life control.

Regular Checkups

Checking on your health: Finding underlying problems like nutrient deficits or long-term illnesses early lets you take action quickly to boost immunity.

Talk to Professionals: Ask your doctor or nurse about personalized immune-supportive strategies.

When you make these changes to your lifestyle, you can strengthen your immune system, protect your body from outside threats, and feel healthier overall. Each habit works with the others to make a cohesive plan for keeping your immune system strong and healthy.

CHAPTER 13

EMOTIONAL WELL-BEING AND CELLULAR HEALTH

Our feelings significantly influence our health when it comes to the cells in our bodies. Being emotionally healthy is important for cell function and overall health. This chapter looks into the mind-body connection and the complex link between emotional health and cellular activity. It also gives useful tips for building emotional resilience.

How Emotional Health Impacts Cellular Function

The state of your emotions has a big impact on the way cells work, both directly and by changing the setting in which cells work. Emotions influence the functioning of cells, either by enhancing their strength and health, or by hindering their healing process and causing dysfunction. When people understand this link, they can take action to support cellular health through mental health.

The Chemical and Emotional Loop

Emotions are not vague; they are based on biology. Hormones, neurotransmitters, and inflammatory markers are like messages that tell cells how to react to our emotions.

Emotional Triggers and Cellular Messaging

Neurological Signals: When you are happy or stressed, your brain sends signals through your nervous system. These signals trigger the release of chemicals such as cortisol, while happiness triggers the release of endorphins. These messages have an effect on how cells make energy, fix them, and protect themselves.

Pathways that cause inflammation: Negative feelings, especially those that last a long time, set off pathways that make inflammatory markers

220

like interleukin-6 (IL-6) and tumor necrosis factor-alpha (TNF-α)
higher. This damages cells.

Oxidative Stress from Negative Emotions

Over time, experiencing negative emotions can increase your body's
production of reactive oxygen species (ROS), potentially leading to
oxidative stress. This can harm the DNA, proteins, and lipids inside
cells. Accelerate mitochondrial malfunction to reduce energy
production. Make it harder for the cell to clean up and fix itself.

Emotional Patterns and Cellular Adaptation

Cells are not static; they adapt to the information they receive. Long-
term emotional stress or negative patterns can alter cellular activity.
On the other hand, positive emotional habits help cells heal and
become stronger.

Emotional Stress and the Aging of Cells

- *Changes in epigenetics:* Long-term stress can alter the expression
  of genes controlling inflammation, metabolism, and aging
  through epigenetic processes. For instance, changes that happen
  because of worry might turn off genes that are in charge of fixing
  DNA.
- *Telomere Erosion:* Stress can very easily damage telomeres,
  which are the caps that protect the ends of chromosomes. Short
  telomeres are associated with faster aging, reduced cell division,
  and an increased risk of illness.

Positive Emotions and Cellular Regeneration

Good emotions like gratitude, kindness, and joy release hormones like
oxytocin and serotonin. Those chemicals are:

- Encourage a cellular setting that reduces inflammation.
- Improve the function of mitochondria, which makes energy
  generation more efficient.
- Start the repair process, which makes cells stronger.

The Role of Emotional Cycles in Circadian Rhythms

Taking care of your emotional health can help keep your body's natural circadian rhythms in balance. These rhythms are important for energy management and cell repair.

Stress and Circadian Disruption

- Chronic worry throws off the hypothalamic-pituitary-adrenal (HPA) axis, which controls the release of cortisol and sleep-wake cycles.
- When circadian rhythms aren't regular, cellular processes like autophagy (cleaning of cells) and mitophagy (removing damaged mitochondria) don't work as well.

Positive Emotions and Circadian Alignment

- Feelings of happiness and calmness control the production of melatonin, a hormone that helps you sleep well and fix cells properly while you're resting.
- Being emotionally stable helps keep cellular clocks in sync across tissues, which speeds up metabolism and lowers stress on cell systems.

Emotional Health and Immune Cells

Emotions have a big effect on the immune system, and immune cells are the first ones to respond to changes in mood.

- ### Chronic Emotional Stress Weakens Immunity

- Over time, high amounts of cortisol slow down the activity of T-cells and natural killer cells. This makes it harder for the body to fight infections and fix damaged cells.
- Chronic negativity can lower the number of lymphocytes in the body, making it more likely to get long-term illnesses that put stress on cell systems.

Positive Emotional Impact on Immunity

Feeling positive makes defense cells work better and more efficiently. As an example: Macrophages, which are cells that eat and kill germs, work more when you're feeling good.

Cytotoxic T-cells work better because they can target and kill sick or damaged cells more effectively.

The Effects of Emotional Patterns over Time

At the cellular level, emotional patterns either hurt or strengthen cells over time.

Prolonged Negative Emotional States

Over time, cells exposed to chronic negative emotions:

- Become less effective at reacting to damage, leading to mutations and cellular senescence (aging).
- Increase the production of molecules that trigger inflammation, thereby placing stress on nearby cells and organs.

The Resilience of Positive Emotional States

Consistent positive emotions encourage:

- The ability of cells to adapt means that they can better handle stress and heal from damage.
- Improved Cell Communication: Release of hormones and neurotransmitters during positive emotions enhances cell communication, facilitating rapid repair and growth.

Practical Takeaways

1. Monitor your mood patterns and regularly consider your mental health. Realizing that negativity lasts for a long time can lead to actions that stop cellular pressure.

2. Do things that make you feel positive about yourself emotionally. Writing in a gratitude book or meditating on the present moment can lower cortisol levels, reduce inflammation, and help cells live longer.

3. Use routines to help you feel emotionally stable: Daily habits that are beneficial for your mental health, like affirmations in the morning or thoughts at night, help keep cellular processes stable.

4. Include playfulness and laughter. Real moments of joy and laughing help cells heal and make mitochondria work better.

5. Help with emotional healing: If you have unresolved emotional damage or long-term stress, getting therapy or counseling can help your cells heal over time.

By combining physical and mental health, you build a base for cell repair, growth, and resilience that supports long-term health.

The Mind-Body Connection and Cellular Repair

There is a close connection between the mind and body. They work together as a dynamic system, and mental states can directly affect how cells work. This link shows how important mental and emotional health is for helping cells heal, grow, and stay healthy generally. By learning about the paths that connect the mind to cellular function, people can take action to improve the health and resilience of their cells.

How do the Mind and Body Communicate?

The nervous, endocrine, and immune systems are just a few of the many signaling systems that make up the mind-body link. These systems turn mental and emotional states into physical reactions that change the way cells work.

What the Nervous System does

Through the nerve system, the brain and spinal cord talk to all the cells in the body. Mental and emotional states, such as worry or relaxation, influence these words.

- Stress Response: Stress activates your sympathetic nervous system (SNS), releasing adrenaline and cortisol. These hormones change the metabolism of cells, the immune system, and the repair process. They often put energy use ahead of healing.
- Relaxation Response: Relaxation or meditation activates your parasympathetic nervous system (PNS). This system lowers cortisol and improves circulation, which helps cells heal, digestion, and immune function.

Hormonal Signaling

Hormones are important because they send messages from the brain to the body's cells. Emotional states affect the production of hormones:

- Feeling positive makes growth hormones and chemicals that help the body heal come out, such as oxytocin.
- Long-term worry raises cortisol, which can stop DNA repair processes, make wounds take longer to heal, and speed up the aging process of cells.

The Role of the Gut-Brain Axis

The gut bacteria and the vagus nerve connect the gut to the brain. This connection has an impact on the health of cells.

- Stress can alter the gut bacteria, exacerbating inflammation and complicating the absorption of nutrients necessary for cell healing.
- Healthy gut bacteria help make neurotransmitters like serotonin, which improve how cells talk to each other and heal.

The Influence of Emotions on Cellular Repair

Depending on how you feel, your emotions can either help or hurt the healing of cells.

Positive Emotions and Healing

- Endorphins and Dopamine: Feelings of happiness and thanks make endorphins and dopamine come out. These chemicals help cells make more energy, make the defense system work better, and speed up the process of fixing DNA.
- Reduces inflammation: Feeling good lowers the production of cytokines that cause inflammation, making the perfect setting for cell recovery.

Negative Emotions and Damage

- More oxidative stress: Long-lasting negative feelings like anger or anxiety make oxidative stress worse by making more reactive oxygen species (ROS). This hurts DNA, proteins, and membranes, which are all parts of cells.
- Mitochondrial Function Problems: Stress that lasts for a long time makes mitochondria less efficient, which means they make less energy, and recovery takes longer.

Neuroplasticity and Cellular Adaptation

Neuroplasticity is the mind's ability to change and adjust. It significantly impacts the health of cells. This adaptability lets people change their mental habits on purpose, creating conditions for cells that help them heal.

- Mindfulness Practices: Regular mindfulness meditation can lower the stress reaction and raise the levels of genes that help cells heal and reduce inflammation.
- Positive Thought Patterns: Studies have shown that cultivating gratitude, positivity, and self-compassion enhances telomerase activity. Telomerase is an enzyme that helps DNA stay safe and cells live longer.

The Science behind the Mind-Body Repair Connection

A new study strongly suggests that the mind can affect the processes of cell repair.

The Role of Telomeres

The caps known as telomeres, which protect chromosomes, are highly sensitive to changes in mental and emotional states.

- Stress and Telomere Shortening: Long-term stress speeds up telomere shortening, which makes cells live shorter and less able to divide and heal themselves.
- Positive Emotions and Telomere Preservation: Studies have demonstrated that meditation, gratitude, and maintaining strong social ties can slow down telomere shortening and even increase telomerase activity.

Epigenetics and Emotional States

Through epigenetic processes, emotional states can change how genes are expressed:

- Stress can turn on genes that cause inflammation and turn off genes that help the body heal itself.
- Having a positive mood can change epigenetic markers, which in turn increases the production of genes that help cells grow, repair, and stay strong.

Brain-Derived Neurotrophic Factor (BDNF)

BDNF is a protein that helps neurons stay alive and heal. BDNF levels rise when you do things that make you feel positive emotionally, like working out and meditating. This helps nerve cells heal and supports the health of all cells.

Practical Strategies for Leveraging the Mind-Body Connection

Start Practicing Mindfulness.

Mindfulness meditation on a regular basis can help control stress hormones, lower inflammation, and create an environment in cells that is beneficial for healing. Aim for 10–20 minutes every day to see changes in your stress levels and the way your cells work.

Work on Controlling your Emotions.

Writing in a journal, cognitive-behavioral therapy (CBT), or doing hobbies can help you deal with negative feelings and boost your positive mood. Mental intelligence training makes relationships and mental strength better, which indirectly benefits cell health.

Make your Social Connections Stronger.

Positive social interactions raise oxytocin levels, lower cortisol levels, and boost immune system function. All of these things help cells heal. Spending time with supportive friends, family, or neighborhood groups on a regular basis can significantly improve your mental health.

Engage in Deep Relaxation Techniques

Practices such as progressive muscle relaxation, yoga, and guided thought activate the parasympathetic nervous system. This makes the perfect environment for cells to heal. Deep breathing exercises can quickly lower your stress and help your cells get more air.

Encourage Thankfulness and Happiness

Practicing gratitude every day, like writing down three things you're grateful for, can change the way your brain works to make it more positive. This can help balance hormones and repair cells. Being optimistic has been linked to less inflammation and better cell health in general.

The mind-body link is a powerful way to help cells heal and become stronger. By focusing on positive emotions, reducing stress, and promoting mental health, individuals can create a biological environment that supports cellular health. Adding these habits to your daily routine builds a basis for long-term health and vitality at the cellular level.

Cultivating Emotional Resilience for Optimal Health

Emotional resilience is the mental and emotional health that comes from being able to deal with stress, problems, and difficulties. This toughness has a direct effect on the health of cells by lowering inflammation, reducing the effects of stress on the body, and helping the body heal and grow. To become emotionally resilient, you need to do more than just be mentally tough. You also need to form habits and ways of thinking that protect and support your body at the cellular level.

Why Emotional Resilience Matters for Cellular Health

Lessening stress: Being emotionally strong helps people deal with stress better, which stops the hypothalamic-pituitary-adrenal (HPA) axis from being overactive all the time. Stress that lasts for a long time can raise cortisol levels and cause oxidative stress and inflammation. All of these things make it harder for cells to work and for DNA to fix itself.

Less inflammation: Resilient individuals experience fewer emotional breakdowns and are less emotionally exhausted, which contributes to a reduction in the production of cytokines that cause inflammation. Lower amounts of inflammation make it easier for cells to repair themselves and grow back.

Better Hormonal Balance: Being emotionally strong helps keep hormones like serotonin, adrenaline, and cortisol stable. This balance is important for things like making energy in mitochondria, keeping the immune system healthy, and cleaning out cells.

Support for neuroplasticity: Being resilient makes the brain more flexible, which supports neuroplasticity. This ability to change helps the brain and body talk to each other better, which is important for keeping cells healthy and supporting long-term vitality.

Important Parts of Being Emotionally Strong

Knowing Yourself

- Becoming resilient starts with understanding your feelings
- Being self-aware helps you figure out what stresses you out and how to deal with it, which stops long-term cellular stress.
- Practice: Writing in a journal or meditating on the present moment can help you become more self-aware by letting you think about your emotional habits.

Optimism and Positive Outlook

- Being optimistic is a key part of being strong. It helps people see problems as chances to learn and grow.
- Studies have linked optimism to lower levels of stress hormones and higher levels of molecules like telomerase that aid in cell repair.
- Practice: Write down things you're thankful for or do visualization techniques to feel better.

Controlling your emotions

- People who are resilient can control their emotions well, which means that negative emotions like anger or worry have less of an effect on their bodies.
- Deep breathing, progressive muscle relaxation, and being aware are all techniques that can help keep your emotions in check.
- When you're feeling stressed, use the 4-7-8 breathing method to quickly lower your cortisol levels.

Problem-Solving Skills

- Being resilient means dealing with problems in a useful way instead of giving up when things get tough.
- You can avoid the feeling of helplessness that makes stress worse by taking steps to solve problems.
- Do it: Break problems down into steps that you can handle, and focus on the answers instead of the problems themselves.

Social Support

- Emotional strength depends on having strong relationships with other people. Cell damage and shorter telomeres are associated with loneliness, but supportive relationships can alleviate loneliness.
- Practice: Make and keep in touch with friends, family, or neighborhood groups that can support and understand you.

Adaptability

- People who are resilient are adaptable and can handle changes in their lives without hurting their physical or mental health.
- Practice: Shift your perspective to view failures as opportunities for growth and avoid adopting rigid thought patterns.

Strategies to Build Emotional Resilience

Develop a Regular Mindfulness Practice

Research demonstrates that mindfulness meditation enhances emotional regulation, reduces stress, and enhances overall strength. It makes you feel relaxed, helps your brain change, and speeds up the healing of cells.

- Start by meditating for 10 minutes every day with a guide.
- Focus on your breath or a certain feeling, and don't judge your ideas as they come and go.

Learn to be Thankful

Being grateful alters the brain's functioning, enhancing its positivity and emotional strength by reducing worry and feelings of lack.

- Every day, write down three things you're thankful for.
- When things are stressful, think about times when you felt joyful and grateful.

Prioritize Sleep and Nutrition

Diet and sleep are essential for mental strength because they keep hormones stable and give the body the energy it needs to respond in a healthy way.

- Aim for 7–8 hours of adequate sleep every night to help your body heal and process emotions.
- Eat foods that are high in antioxidants, omega-3 fatty acids, and B vitamins. These foods are beneficial for your brain and mental health.

Do Regular Physical Activities

Get some exercise to reduce stress, boost happiness, and release endorphins, which strengthen your emotions.

- Do gentle exercise for at least 30 minutes most days of the week.
- Do things like yoga, which combine being aware and moving.

Engage in Cognitive Behavioral Therapy (CBT) Techniques

Cognitive behavioral therapy (CBT) can help you change negative thought habits into helpful ones. This boosts resilience and reduces cell damage from stress.

- Write down your thoughts so you can question harmful ones and replace them with more balanced ones.

- Say positive affirmations to yourself every day to keep your strong attitude.

Connect with Nature

The mind and body feel better after spending time in nature. It lowers cortisol levels and helps keep emotions in check.

- Go for walks or "forest bathing" in green areas every day for 20 to 30 minutes.
- Do things outside, like gardening, to relax and get some exercise.

The Role of Resilience in Cellular Health

Building emotional strength isn't just a mental workout; it also has real health benefits for cells. When someone is resilient, they make their body's cells less vulnerable to harmful stress chemicals, inflammation, and oxidative stress. This helps with:

- Improved mitochondrial function provides cells with the necessary energy to grow and repair themselves.
- Turning on DNA repair systems slows down cell harm over time.
- Made the immune system work better, which keeps cells safe from infections and long-term illnesses.

Building mental strength is an important part of keeping cells healthy. You can protect your cells from the damage of chronic stress and create a healthy, healing environment inside your body by improving your ability to deal with life's difficulties. You can build resilience through techniques like mindfulness, gratitude, and effective stress management. This will not only improve your mental health but also your cells' long-term health and vitality.

CHAPTER 14

CREATING A CELLULAR HEALTH ROUTINE FOR LONG-TERM VITALITY

Setting up a habit that puts cellular health first is important for staying healthy over time. This chapter covers how to make lifelong habits that improve cell health, track your success, and have daily habits that improve cell health. Living by these rules can give you more energy, slow down the aging process, and make your health better in general.

How to Build a Daily Habit for Cellular Well-Being

To support cellular health every day, you need to do things on purpose, consistently, and in different ways that help your body fix, renew, and protect itself at the cellular level. Establishing these habits may seem challenging, but by taking strategic steps, you can establish a lifestyle that prioritizes cellular health that will last.

The first step is to figure out what your cell phone needs are. Micronutrients, like vitamins and minerals, and macronutrients, like carbs, proteins, and fats, are what cells need to make energy, fix damage, and keep doing their jobs. Staying hydrated is an important part of cellular metabolism and cleansing. Exercise increases blood flow, which brings oxygen and nutrients to cells. Cellular repair and renewal also depend on rest and healing, such as getting enough sleep and dealing with stress. Once you understand these basic needs, you can establish habits that regularly meet them.

Keeping things simple and doable should always be your top concern. It's challenging to stick to complicated habits, so starting with small steps that you can do can make a big difference. Having a glass of water first thing in the morning can help your cells get back to normal after a night's sleep. Adding one nutrient-dense food to each meal, like nuts or fresh greens, can help you get a lot more nutrients. Reminding yourself to take breaks to move, such as stretching or walking, every hour will help you stay active. Consistency is much more important over time than trying to be perfect every once in a while, so keep your schedule simple and straightforward to handle.

Another successful method is to set up a habit loop. There is a cue, a pattern, and a reward in a habit loop. Putting a water bottle on your nightstand can remind you to do healthy things, like drinking water first thing in the morning. Consistently following the cue, like stretching for five minutes right after getting up, forms the habit. Giving yourself a reward for doing something, like noticing how energized you feel, helps the habit stick over time. These cues and benefits build neural pathways that make the habit happen on its own.

Making a habit that focuses on cellular health can make your health a lot better. You might drink 16–20 ounces of water in the morning, mixing it with lemon to add antioxidants. Then, you might eat a breakfast that is high in protein, healthy fats, and antioxidants to power mitochondrial energy production. Lifting light weights or going for a quick walk can wake up your muscles and cells. You could have a balanced lunch with lean proteins, complex carbohydrates, and colorful vegetables in the middle of the day for long-lasting energy. During this time, you could also practice mindfulness through deep breathing or writing in a gratitude journal to lower stress, and take five-minute movement breaks every hour to prevent cellular stagnation. Focusing on an anti-inflammatory dinner with whole grains, cruciferous veggies, and omega-3-rich proteins in the evening is a beneficial idea. Limiting screen time an hour before bed helps your body make melatonin, and a relaxing wind-down process gets your body ready to repair and regenerate itself overnight.

Keeping track of your work and thinking about it helps you stay going. You can keep track of things like how much water you drink, how much exercise you do, and the quality of your meals by using habit trackers, which can be apps or real charts. Writing in a journal about how these habits affect your health, happiness, and energy can help you learn a lot. You can use biometrics such as energy levels, skin quality, and sleep habits to assess the health of your cells and identify areas for improvement.

Being flexible is important for getting past problems. Life is unpredictable, and staying healthy at the cellular level means being able to change. You can bring healthy snacks with you, drink water, and do short stretches while you're moving. For people with busy lives, nutrient-dense, ready-made foods or short, intense workouts work well. To be aware, choose vegetables, lean proteins, and water over processed foods and sugary drinks when you're with other people.

Support and responsibility can make it much easier to stick to healthy habits for cells. Talking about your goals with family and friends, getting personalized help from a nutritionist or fitness coach, or joining neighborhood groups that focus on healthy living can help you stay motivated and learn from each other.

A strong motivation is to think about how good habits for cellular health will help you in the long run. Doing things over and over again gives you more energy, makes you stronger, lowers your chance of getting chronic diseases, and improves your quality of life in general. Visualizing these results can help you stay committed.

Change your habit to help you grow as your needs change. Check in with your goals every so often to make sure your habits are helping you reach them. Adding variety to your routine, like switching up meals, exercises, and ways to relax, makes it interesting. Celebrating small wins, like having more energy or sleeping better, helps keep the work going.

To make a daily habit for cellular health, you need to be aware, consistent, and able to change your mind. Creating habits that put hydration, nutrition, movement, and recovery at the top of the list will help your cells grow. These habits become second nature over time, creating a way of life that supports long-term health and strength.

Tracking Your Progress: Metrics and Strategies

Keeping track of your progress is important for staying motivated, figuring out what's working, and making the changes you need to make to improve your cells' health. When you combine objective data with subjective feedback, you can get a full picture of how your habits are affecting your health at the cellular level. This method gives you the power to stay constant and find long-term health.

Why Keep Track of Your Progress?

Tracking gives you useful information about your path to better cell health. It assists you in identifying the habits that are beneficial to you and those that may require modification. It keeps you inspired by showing you real progress and holds you more accountable, which helps you stick to your goals. Tracking is also a form of preventative care because it helps you find early signs of possible health problems.

Key Metrics for Healthy Cells

It's crucial to concentrate on measurable results and visible health changes when monitoring your cellular health. To give you an example, your energy levels show exactly how healthy your mitochondria are. Low energy all the time could mean that you aren't getting enough to eat, rest, or protect yourself from toxic stress. You can keep track of this by giving your daily energy levels a score from 1 to 10 and writing down any trends or drops you notice during the day.

Another important sign is the quality of your sleep, which is a big part of fixing cells and getting rid of toxins. You can monitor this by monitoring the number of hours you sleep (ideally 7–9 hours), tracking your sleep cycles using smart tech or apps, and assessing how rested you feel upon waking up.

The health of your skin and hair shows how well your cells are healing and getting water. Taking pictures of your skin every week can help you see changes in tone, flexibility, moisture, or shine. Digestive health holds significant importance as it influences the functioning of cells and the absorption of nutrients. Writing down your bowel movement habits, bloating, or pain in a journal can help you find important trends.

Another important measure is immune resilience, since a strong immune system means that cells can communicate and repair themselves well. Keeping track of how often you get sick or how long it takes to get better can show that your immune system is getting stronger. Blood markers like glucose and cholesterol levels, as well as biometrics like body composition, resting heart rate, and blood pressure, give clear information on the health of cells.

Subjective Feedback

Subjective feedback goes along with objective metrics and gives you a more personal look at your general health. Keeping track of changes in your mood, mental clarity, and emotional stability can help you see how far you've come. Keeping track of how stressed you feel, how your food habits change, and how long it takes you to recover from exercise can also show that your health and cell repair are getting better.

Tools and Strategies for Tracking

Tools like journals, apps, and smart tech are very helpful for keeping track of your progress. You can keep track of your happiness, energy levels, meals, exercise, and sleep quality by writing in a journal. Apps like MyFitnessPal and Fitbit provide real-time access to health, exercise, and heart rate data. Wearables give you more information about how you sleep and how active you are. By comparing photos of your skin, hair, and stance on a regular basis, you can see small changes that happen over time.

Going over your data once a week or once a month can help you think about your progress and make plans for the next time, such as setting new goals or making changes.

Tips for Being Consistent

Consistency in tracking is important for getting enough information to make smart choices. You can keep up with the habit by setting reminders, making tracking a part of your daily life, and enjoying small wins like more energy or better digestion.

Recognizing and Addressing Plateaus

If you encounter a plateau in your progress, examine your habits and ensure you maintain essential ones such as maintaining proper hydration, maintaining a healthy diet, and getting adequate sleep. To break out of a rut, reevaluate your goals or vary your daily routine. You might also find it helpful to talk to a doctor or chef about how to improve your approach.

How Tracking Can Lead to Long-Term Success

Keeping track of your progress sets off a feedback loop that pushes you to keep getting better. By keeping track of what works and changing your habits and routines, you can create a long-term way of life that supports the health of your cells. As you do this regularly, you will be able to fine-tune your efforts, enjoy your successes, and get past problems. This will help you build a routine that supports your cells' health and strength.

Developing Lifelong Healthy Habits

To achieve ongoing vitality and cellular well-being, it is essential to form and stick to healthy habits that will last a lifetime. Making short-term changes can help, but making habits a part of your daily life will keep your body healthy on a cellular level. To keep up healthy habits over time, you don't need to take drastic steps. Instead, you should take a slow, steady approach that fits your wants and way of life.

The Importance of Sustainability in Health Habits

Sustainability is crucial for long-term success because too strict or difficult-to-maintain habits often lead to loops of inconsistency. Sustainable habits help you keep getting better and make sure your body gets regular care, which is important for cell regrowth. Daily actions that are simple to handle are better for your general health than short bursts of hard work. Also, long-lasting habits lower stress, which is beneficial for your mental and emotional health and keeps you motivated and in control.

Key Principles for Building Sustainable Health Habits

To make healthy habits that last a lifetime, it's best to begin small and build up over time. Lots of changes at once can be challenging to handle, so start with a few simple ones, like drinking more water or going for a short walk after meals. You can gradually add small changes over time. For example, you could eat more fruits and veggies or do deep breathing exercises.

Being consistent is more important than being perfect. Progress is not always linear, and striving for perfection can lead to frustration. Instead, focus on regularly making small, beneficial choices, even if you have setbacks now and then. Do not judge your success as you track it; celebrate small wins to keep yourself going.

Making habits fun makes them more likely to last. It's easier to stick to healthy habits when you do things you enjoy, like dancing, hiking, or trying new foods. It can be more enjoyable and interesting to share your journey with a health buddy or a group.

Habits have meaning when they are in line with your values and goals. Think about why you want to improve the health of your cells—maybe to feel more energized, live longer, or feel less stressed—and connect your habits to those goals. Focusing on sleep and anti-inflammatory foods can feel meaningful and motivating if you want to live a long time.

Making habits simple makes them simpler to follow through with. To make healthy choices easier, plan your meals, lay out your workout clothes the night before, or get rid of obstacles.

How Can You Maintain Your Motivation Over Time?

Maintaining healthy habits requires consistent effort. Keeping track of success with journals, apps, or photos shows that things are getting better, like better sleep or glowing skin. Acknowledging small victories, such as working out every day for a month, keeps you motivated and prevents burnout.

Your habits can change with the times if you stay open with them. If you don't have much time, shorter workouts or meals that are easier to make can help you stay on track. You'll stay on track if you change how you do things instead of giving up habits.

Getting Through Challenges

Because life is unpredictable, problems will always come up, but if you deal with them early on, you can avoid mistakes. For instance, if cooking every day seems like too much work, making meals ahead of time or picking simple recipes can help. Being resilient also means seeing losses as chances to learn instead of as failures. If you miss a workout, reflect on why you missed it and adjust your plan to make it easier to maintain. Seeking assistance from a health coach, an online community, or a friend who shares your objectives can ensure your accountability and provide support during challenging times.

Incorporate Cell-Healthy Habits into your Everyday Routine.

For habits to last, they need to fit in with your daily life without any problems. This means making healthy meals a normal part of your day while still giving yourself some freedom so that eating well doesn't feel like a chore. Making meals ahead of time makes sure that there are always healthy choices.

You should pick workouts that you enjoy and that help you reach your goals, like dancing, yoga, or power training. Making plans for workouts ahead of time can help you make them a normal part of your life. Having a happy attitude by practicing gratitude and doing stress-relieving activities like deep breathing or meditation every day is also good for your emotional and mental health.

To make healthy habits that last a lifetime, you need to set reasonable goals, be consistent, and be open to change. You can set yourself up for long-term success by starting small, making habits fun, making sure they are in line with your values, and staying motivated. Keeping track of your success and overcoming problems will help you stay committed to your health goals. Integrating these habits into your daily life will ultimately help your cells stay healthy and strong.

CONCLUSION

RECLAIMING YOUR VITALITY – THE PATH TO CELLULAR LONGEVITY

In this series on cellular health, we've looked at the big benefits of feeding your cells the right foods, helping them get rid of toxins, and making the most of cellular repair. Follow the Cellular Health Diet to gain energy, strength, and the tools to restore your health and prolong cell life.

This method isn't just about living longer; it's also about living better. Your body's functions depend on healthy cells, which give you energy, protect you from getting sick, and help you live a full, busy life. Despite the complexity of the science behind cell health, making the necessary changes is straightforward. Small, regular actions that have long-lasting effects over time are the key to optimal health and long-lasting cells.

Here, we'll talk more about how these changes can fit into your life, how important movement is for cellular health, and how you can take charge of your path to lifelong wellness.

Reclaiming Your Vitality – The Path to Cellular Longevity

Vitality is a normal state that your body can reach if you take care of its cells. Your body can move, grow, and do well with healthy cells. You can live a strong and full life by focusing on cellular longevity, which means making sure cells work at their best for as long as possible.

The Link between Healthy Cells and a Longer Life

Aging and maintaining health are closely associated with cellular health. Toxins, inflammation, and oxidative stress are damaging cells over time, which slows down energy production and healing processes. This can lead to chronic diseases and physical decline in the long run.

But you can make changes to your habits that will make your cells live longer, such as eating better, exercising regularly, and dealing with stress better. These changes can:

- Support autophagy, which is the body's natural way of "cleaning up" cells and helping them heal.
- Improve the health of your mitochondria, which will help your body make more energy and feel less tired.
- Lessen inflammation, which lowers the risk of long-term diseases like Alzheimer's, heart disease, and diabetes.
- Maintain DNA integrity, which prevents cell damage that accelerates aging.

The Cellular Health Diet gives you ways to feed and clean out your cells, but exercise is also crucial for improving cellular health.

The Power of Small, Consistent Changes

For the health of cells, consistency is more important than beauty. Small changes made regularly add up over time, causing a chain reaction that improves the health of cells and the body as a whole. One of the most life-changing things you can do is add movement to your daily life.

Movement: A Booster for Cellular Health

Aside from burning calories and growing muscle, exercise has a huge effect on the health of your cells. Here are some of the primary benefits of exercise:

- Better functioning of mitochondria: Exercise raises the amount and effectiveness of mitochondria, which makes your body better able to create energy (ATP). Walking, cycling, and power training are some of the best things you can do.
- Better cellular detoxification: exercise increases circulation and blood flow, which makes it easier for the body to get rid of waste

and toxins. Sweating while you work out helps the body get rid of toxins even more.

- Activation of Autophagy: Exercise speeds up autophagy, which gets rid of broken cell parts and helps cells heal and grow again.
- Less inflammation: Regular exercise lowers the production of pro-inflammatory molecules, which protects cells from damage and slows down the aging process.
- Protecting DNA and telomeres: Exercise helps protect and stretch telomeres, which are the caps that protect DNA and slow down the aging process.

Incorporating Movement into Your Lifestyle

Active movement benefits your health without spending hours at the gym. Finding enjoyable things to do that fit easily into your daily life is the key. Start slowly by doing something like swift walking, stretching, or dancing for 10 to 15 minutes. As you become accustomed to it, extend the duration. Find things you love doing, like gardening, yoga, swimming, or your favorite sport, and make moving around a pleasure instead of a chore.

Do strength training workouts two to three times a week. You can use your own body weight, dumbbells, or resistance bands. Not only does this build muscle, it also makes mitochondria work better. Intensity is not as important as consistency. Short, regular sessions are better for cell health than random, powerful ones. Aim for 30 minutes of moderate exercise most days and move around a lot during the day. Instead of taking the lift, take the stairs. While on the phone, walk around. Or, take five-minute breaks every hour to move around.

In addition to regular exercise, restorative moves like yoga, tai chi, or stretching can help lower stress, increase flexibility, and speed up cell repair by calming the nervous system.

You can improve the health of your cells and set yourself up for a life of lasting energy and resilience by making movement a priority along with a healthy diet and regular self-care.

Your Journey to Optimal Health and Resilience

Your path to better health is unique. Discover what works for you and embrace change. It's not about having a strict set of rules. For your reference, here are some rules to follow:

Progress, Not Perfection

When making life changes, you may feel stressed. Don't forget that the goal is growth, not perfection. Add more veggies to your meals or go for a 10-minute walk after dinner. These are all small steps that you can easily take.

Listen to Your Body

Your body is always telling you what it wants. Pay attention to how you feel after you eat certain things, work out, or deal with worry. Now that you know this, change your habits and make a pattern that feels beneficial and will last.

Stay Flexible and Adapt

Because life is unpredictable, there will be times when it's challenging to stick to a plan. Be kind to yourself and change when you need to. The most important thing is that you want to get back on track.

Enjoy the Little Wins.

You should be proud of every step you take to improve your health. Whether it's getting more water, sleeping better, or working out for the first time, celebrate your progress and use it to keep going.

Final Words of Encouragement for Lifelong Wellness

Remember that you are empowered to change your life as you start this journey to get your energy back and put cellular health first. Your cells are strong and flexible, and they can heal, grow, and fix themselves with the right help.

Choosing nutrient-dense foods, moving your body, or dealing with stress are all small changes that add up over time to make you healthy and more vibrant. It might not always be easy, but the trip is very worth it.

It's your turn now. Now is the time to take charge of your health, feel strong and energized, and live a full, healthy life. Trust the process and start from where you are. You can accomplish great things and live a healthy life.

One last call to action

Tell us about your trip. Motivate people by setting a positive example. The choices you make today affect more than just your health. They will also affect the health of your friends, family, and future generations, inspiring them to put cellular health and life first.

Let this be the start of a life full of joy, energy, and strength. Get your energy back, and then firmly move into the future you deserve.